A Workbook of Manual Therapy Techniques

A Workbook of Manual Therapy Techniques for the Vertebral Column and Pelvic Girdle

Diane G. Lee B.S.R., M.C.P.A., C.O.M.P.
Instructor, Orthopaedic Division, C.P.A.
Examiner, Canadian Orthopaedic Manipulative Physiotherapists

Mari C. Walsh M.C.S.P., M.C.P.A., C.O.M.P.
Instructor, Orthopaedic Division, C.P.A.

ISBN 0-88925-639-X

Published by
Nacent Publishing
302-8425 120th St.,Delta B.C. V4C 6R2
Canada

Second printing, 1991

Printed and bound in Canada by
Friesen Printers
a Division of D. W. Friesen & Sons Ltd.
Head Office
Altona, Manitoba R0G 0B0
Canada

Dedication
To Michael
– another new beginning

PREFACE

Musculoskeletal disorders can be effectively treated with physiotherapy, including mobilization (active and passive), stabilization,
electrotherapy, thermotherapy, cryotherapy and education. Manual therapy
is one method of mobilization and refers to treatment which requires the use
of one's hands – aside from applying machinery! Although the definition is
broad, manual therapy is a small part of physiotherapy and is only as
effective as the ability to accurately detect the dysfunction for which it is
indicated.

The intent of this workbook is to assist the student in acquiring the skills
of manual therapy for the vertebral column and pelvic girdle both in examination and treatment technique by detailed exposition and illustration. The
techniques outlined in this workbook are not meant to be exclusive of all
others, but are rather a solid base from which the learning therapist can
expand. It is hoped that this workbook will be used as an adjunct to the
Canadian Orthopaedic Manipulative Therapy courses, part of which
requires the instruction of these examination and treatment techniques.

For the beginner, we have purposely presented the techniques in a
dissected manner recognizing that the skilled clinician may view this dissec-
tion as abuse of the art. Indeed, experience teaches us that dogma and recipes
have no place in the science or the art of manual therapy, however, for each
and everyone of us, there was a beginning.

ACKNOWLEDGEMENTS

We would like to take this opportunity to express our thanks to those without whom this work would have remained just a 'good idea.' Our photographer, Thomas Lee, who not only patiently clicked hundreds of photographs, but withstood the test of yet another physiotherapy project. Our graphic artist, Roland Kirsten, who designed the cover, the dividers and the craniovertebral line diagrams. Our models, Grant Gibson and Carolann Jakeman, our typist, Stacy Flatt. Special thanks to R.R. Roman. And last, but certainly not least, our colleagues, from whom many of these techniques are derived, a constant source of support, enthusiasm and ideas.

We would also like to acknowledge Churchill Livingstone for their kind permission to reproduce the figures on pages xv, 98, 100, orginally drawn by Alun Morgan.

TABLE OF CONTENTS

Treatment

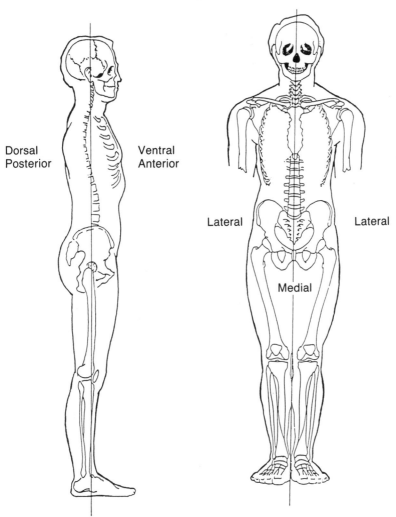

Cranial

Dorsal
Posterior

Ventral
Anterior

Lateral

Lateral

Medial

Caudal

Definition of Direction

Craniovertebral Region

Occipito–atlantal and Atlanto–axial Joints

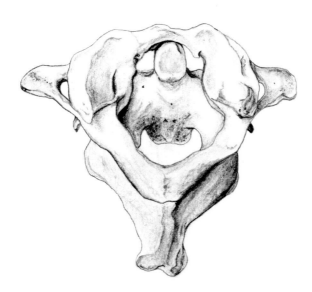

Craniovertebral Region — Occipito-atlantal and Atlanto-axial Joints

1. POSITIONAL TESTS

    a) Occipito–atlantal joints (O/A)

Patient:	Supine, head supported on a pillow.
Therapist:	Standing at the patient's head facing the shoulders.
Palpate:	With the index fingers, palpate the distance between the transverse process of the atlas and the mastoid process of the temporal bone bilaterally. Compare the left to the right side. The side to which the occiput is sideflexed is the side of the shortest distance.

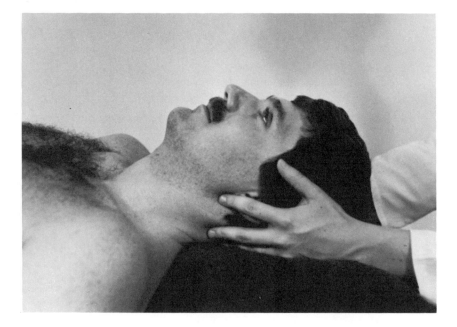

Notes:

_____

_____

_____

_____

_____

_____

_____

_____

_____

_____

_____

_____

_____

_____

_____

_____

_____

_____

_____

_____

_____

2. MOBILITY TESTS – Specific Articular Mobility

a) Occipito–atlantal joints (O/A)

1. Flexion/Extension

Patient: Supine, head supported on a pillow.

Therapist: Standing at the patient's head facing the shoulders.

Palpate: With the index fingers, palpate the mastoid process of the temporal bone bilaterally. The rest of the hand supports the cranium.

Test: Passively or actively flex/extend the O/A joints about a coronal axis through the mastoid processes. Note the quantity and quality of motion.

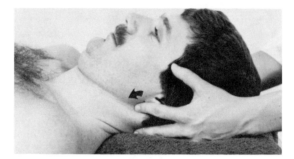

2. Sideflexion/Rotation

Patient: Supine, head supported on a pillow.

Therapist: Standing at the patient's head facing the shoulders.

Palpate: With the index fingers, palpate the mastoid process of the temporal bone bilaterally.

Test: Passively sideflex the O/A joints about a sagittal axis through the nose. Rotation occurs in conjunction with sideflexion. Note the quantity and quality of motion.

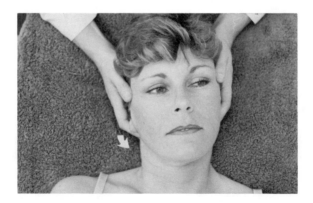

Notes:

_____

_____

_____

_____

_____

_____

_____

_____

_____

_____

_____

_____

_____

_____

_____

_____

_____

_____

_____

_____

2. MOBILITY TESTS — Specific Articular Mobility

b) Atlanto-axial joints (A/A)

1. Flexion/Extension

Patient: Supine, head supported on a pillow.

Therapist: Standing at the patient's head facing the shoulders.

Palpate: With the index fingers, palpate the interspace between the posterior arch of the atlas and the lamina of the axis bilaterally. The rest of the hand supports the cranium.

Test: Passively flex/extend the O/A joints first. Then, passively flex/extend the A/A joints about a coronal axis through the dens. Note the quantity and quality of motion. (See left figure below)

2. Rotation

Patient: Supine, head supported on a pillow.

Therapist: Standing at the patient's head facing the shoulders.

Palpate: With the index and long fingers, palpate the lateral side of the bifid spinous process of the axis bilaterally. The rest of the hand supports the cranium.

Test: *With the O/A and A/A joints in a neutral position,* rotate the A/A joints about a vertical axis until movement of the spinous process of the C2 vertebra is perceived against the index and long fingers. At this point, the total available rotation of the A/A joints has occurred. Note the quantity and quality of motion. (See right figure below)

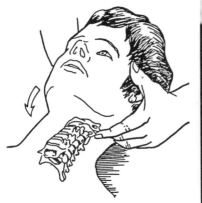 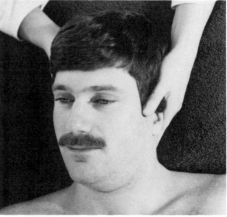

CRANIOVERTEBRAL REGION   ASSESSMENT

Notes:

_____

_____

_____

_____

_____

_____

_____

_____

_____

_____

_____

_____

_____

_____

_____

_____

_____

_____

_____

_____

_____

3. STRESS TESTS

a) Alar Ligaments

Patient:	Sitting or supine.
	N.B. The craniovertebral joints must be in a neutral position.
Therapist:	Standing beside the seated patient or standing at the patient's head facing the shoulders if the patient is supine.
Palpate:	**1. Patient:** Sitting. With the thumb and index/long fingers of the dorsal hand, palpate the spinous process of the C2 vertebra. The ventral hand cups the top of the cranium.
	2. Patient: Supine. With the index and long fingers, palpate the lateral side of the bifid spinous process of the C2 vertebra bilaterally. The rest of the hand supports the cranium.
Test:	Passively sideflex the O/A joints about a sagittal axis through the nose. *Immediate* movement of the spinous process of the C2 vertebra to the opposite side should be felt if the alar ligament contralateral to the side of the sideflexion motion is intact.

Repeat the test to the opposite side.

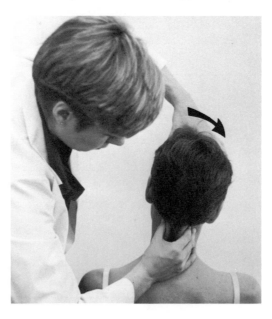

Notes:

_____

_____

_____

_____

_____

_____

_____

_____

_____

_____

_____

_____

_____

_____

_____

_____

_____

_____

_____

_____

_____

_____

3. STRESS TESTS

b) Transverse ligament/dens — ventral

Patient: Supine, head supported on a pillow.

Therapist: Standing at the patient's head facing the shoulders.

Palpate: With the index fingers, palpate transversely the posterior arch of the atlas between the inion and the spinous process of the C2 vertebra. The rest of the hand supports the cranium.

Test: With the index fingers, apply a slow, steady, anterior shear against the posterior arch of the atlas. This is restrained by the osseous integrity of the dens as well as the transverse ligament.

Note the quantity and quality of motion.

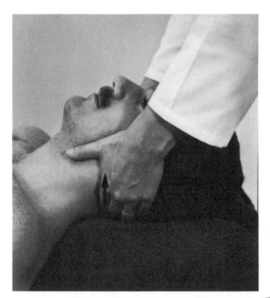

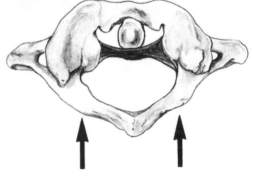

Notes:

_____

_____

_____

_____

_____

_____

_____

_____

_____

_____

_____

_____

_____

_____

_____

_____

_____

_____

_____

_____

_____

CRANIOVERTEBRAL REGION   ASSESSMENT

3. STRESS TESTS

c) Transverse ligament/dens — lateral

Patient: Supine, head supported on a pillow.

Therapist: Standing at the patient's head facing the shoulders.

Palpate: With the lateral aspect of the MCP joint of the right index finger, palpate the right transverse process of the atlas. With the lateral aspect of the MCP joint of the left index finger, palpate the left transverse process of the C2 vertebra.

Test: Fix the atlas with the right hand and attempt to laterally shear the C2 vertebra to the right. Switch hands, fix the atlas on the left and attempt to laterally shear the C2 vertebra to the left. Note the quantity and quality of motion.

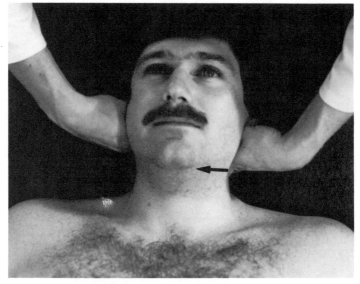

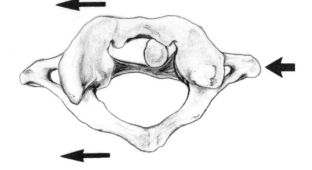

Notes:

_____

_____

_____

_____

_____

_____

_____

_____

_____

_____

_____

_____

_____

_____

_____

_____

_____

_____

_____

_____

_____

_____

4. VERTEBRAL ARTERY TEST

Patient: Supine, without a pillow.

Therapist: Standing at the patient's head facing the shoulders.

Test: Passively extend the cervical spine to the maximum available range. Hold this position for 30 seconds and note any symptoms (dizziness, dysequilibrium, upper or lower quadrant dysaesthesiae) or signs (nystagmus). From this maximally extended position, rotate the cranium to the left. Hold this position for 30 seconds and note any symptoms or signs produced. Rotate the cranium to the right. Hold this position for 30 seconds and note any symptoms or signs produced.

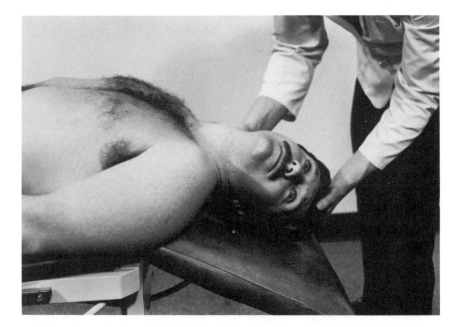

Notes:

_____

_____

_____

_____

_____

_____

_____

_____

_____

_____

_____

_____

_____

_____

_____

_____

_____

_____

_____

_____

_____

_____

_____

1. PASSIVE SOFT TISSUE MOBILIZATION

a) Longitudinal: suboccipital tissue

Patient: Supine, head supported on a pillow.

Therapist: Standing or sitting at the patient's head facing the shoulders.

Palpate: With the forearms supinated and the fingers flexed in a lumbrical grip, palpate the suboccipital tissue bilaterally. The distal $\frac{1}{3}$ of the forearms should be supported on the table.

Mobilization: *Do Not* use the finger flexors. This produces a digging sensation as opposed to an effective stretch. Apply a slow, steady stretch via elbow flexion and release.

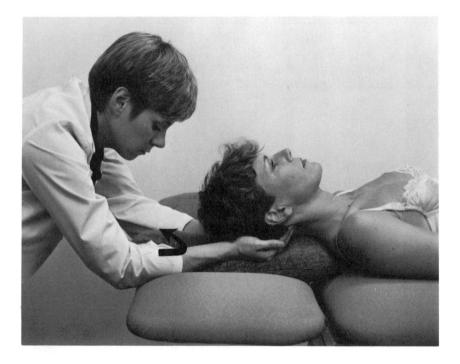

Notes:

_____

_____

_____

_____

_____

_____

_____

_____

_____

_____

_____

_____

_____

_____

_____

_____

_____

_____

_____

_____

_____

1. PASSIVE SOFT TISSUE MOBILIZATION

b) Transverse: suboccipital tissue

Patient: Supine, head supported on a pillow.

Therapist: Standing at the side of the table, level with the patient's cranium.

Palpate: Place the dorsal aspect of the cranial hand against the patient's zygoma. With the index and long fingers of the caudal hand, palpate the posterior arch of the atlas on the opposite side.

Mobilization: Fix the cranium with the cranial hand and apply a slow, steady stretch to the suboccipital tissue by pulling the atlas ventrally and medially.

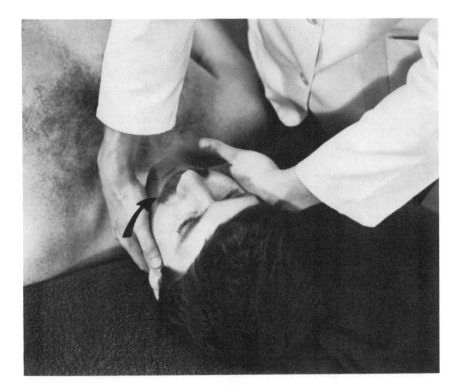

Notes:

_____

_____

_____

_____

_____

_____

_____

_____

_____

_____

_____

_____

_____

_____

_____

_____

_____

_____

_____

_____

_____

_____

2. PASSIVE ARTICULAR MOBILIZATION

a) Occipito-atlantal joints (O/A)

1. Flexion/Extension

Patient: Supine, the presence of a pillow depends on the flexibility of the cervicothoracic junction.

Therapist: Standing at the patient's head facing the shoulders.

Palpate: With the lateral aspect of the MCP joint of the index finger, palpate transversely the posterior arch of the atlas. The ulnar border of this hand rests on the table. With the other hand, cup the occiput.

Mobilization: a) Flexion: Gravity assist. Accessory Glide: allow the occiput to descend dorsally on the fixed atlas. Physiological Movement: physiological flexion can be incorporated by passively flexing the O/A joints as the occiput descends dorsally.

b) Extension: Accessory Glide: glide the occiput in a ventral direction on the atlas. Physiological Movement: physiological extension can be incorporated by passively extending the O/A joints as the occiput glides ventrally.

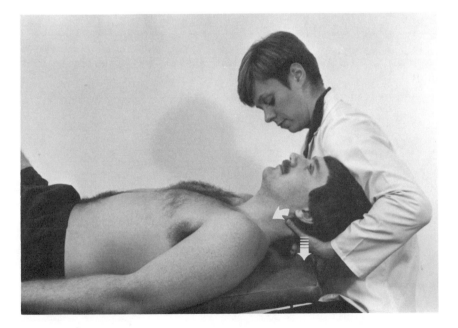

Notes:

_____

_____

_____

_____

_____

_____

_____

_____

_____

_____

_____

_____

_____

_____

_____

_____

_____

_____

_____

_____

_____

_____

2. PASSIVE ARTICULAR MOBILIZATION

   a) Occipito–atlantal joints (O/A)

      2. Sideflexion/Rotation

Patient:	Sitting, spine supported against the chair.
Therapist:	Standing at the patient's side.
Palpate:	With an open pinch grip, palpate the posterior arch of the atlas with the dorsal hand. The cranium is cradled with the ventral hand/arm such that the palmar aspect of the 5th digit is applied to the temporal/occipital region.
Localization:	Fix the atlas and laterally glide the occiput towards the therapist.
Mobilization:	A straight lateral glide of the occiput in the transverse plane towards the therapist reproduces the conjunct glide associated with sideflexion at this level (see photograph). Since physiological sideflexion is conjoined with contralateral rotation, this technique is more effective if the congruent physiological motions are incorporated with the accessory glide. One occipital condyle glides ventromedially on the atlas while the opposite glides dorsolaterally (see diagram).

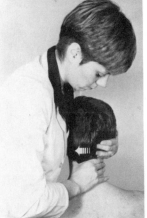

Notes:

_____

_____

_____

_____

_____

_____

_____

_____

_____

_____

_____

_____

_____

_____

_____

_____

_____

_____

_____

_____

_____

_____

2. PASSIVE ARTICULAR MOBILIZATION
  b) Atlanto–axial joints (A/A)
    1. Rotation

Patient: Sitting, spine supported against the chair.

Therapist: Standing at the patient's side.

Palpate: With an open pinch grip of the dorsal hand, palpate the posterior arch of the axis. The ventral hand cradles the cranium such that the palmer aspect of the 5th digit is applied to the posterior arch of the atlas.

Mobilization: Fix the axis and rotate the atlanto–axial joints.

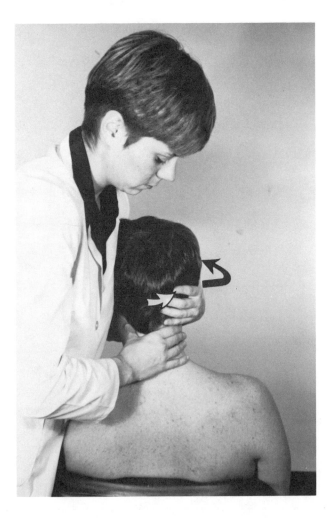

Notes:

_____

_____

_____

_____

_____

_____

_____

_____

_____

_____

_____

_____

_____

_____

_____

_____

_____

_____

_____

_____

_____

_____

3. ACTIVE MOBILIZATION
  a) Occipito–atlantal joints (O/A)
    1. Flexion

Patient:	Supine, the presence of a pillow depends on the flexibility of the cervicothoracic junction.
Therapist:	Standing at the patient's head facing the shoulders.
Palpate:	With the lateral aspect of the MCP joint of the index finger, palpate transversely the posterior arch of the atlas. With the other hand, cup the occiput.
Localization:	The motion barrier is localized by flexing the O/A joints about the appropriate coronal axis to the physiological limit.
Mobilization:	From this position, the patient is instructed to hold the head still while the therapist minimally releases the support of the cranium. This isometric contraction recruits the deep and superficial cervical flexor muscles and is held for 3–5 seconds. Full support is reapplied and the patient is instructed to completely relax. The new flexion barrier is localized. The mobilization is repeated 3 times.
Extension	The technique is identical to the above except that extension is employed instead of flexion.

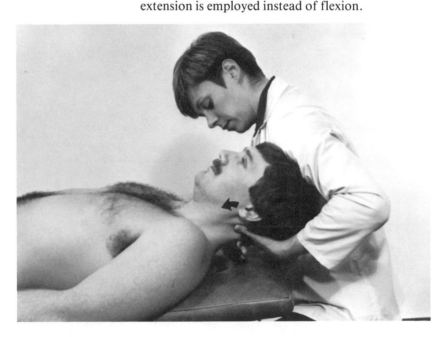

Notes:

_____

_____

_____

_____

_____

_____

_____

_____

_____

_____

_____

_____

_____

_____

_____

_____

_____

_____

_____

_____

_____

3. ACTIVE MOBILIZATION

a) Occipito–atlantal joints (O/A)

2. Flexion/Sideflexion/Rotation

Patient: Supine, head supported on a pillow.

Therapist: Standing at the patient's head facing the shoulders.

Palpate: It is not necessary during active mobilization techniques to rigidly fix the atlas, however, accurate localization of the motion barrier is essential. Therefore, the index fingers palpate the suboccipital space while the rest of the hand supports the cranium.

Localization: The motion barrier is localized by flexing, sideflexing and contralaterally rotating the O/A joints to the physiological limit.

Mobilization: From this position, the patient is instructed to hold the head still while the therapist applies minimal resistance (arrow) to rotation of the cranium. The direction is not significant since myofascial relaxation can occur via both reciprocal or autogenic inhibition. This isometric contraction is held for 3–5 seconds. The resistance is gently released and the patient is instructed to completely relax. The new flexion/sideflexion/rotation barrier is localized. The mobilization is repeated 3 times. (See left figure below)

3. Extension/Sideflexion/Rotation

The technique is identical to the above except that extension is employed instead of flexion. (See right figure below)

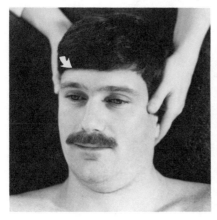 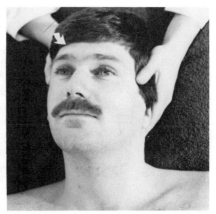

Notes:

_____

_____

_____

_____

_____

_____

_____

_____

_____

_____

_____

_____

_____

_____

_____

_____

_____

_____

_____

_____

_____

_____

3. ACTIVE MOBILIZATION
b) Atlanto–axial joints (A/A)

   1. Rotation

Patient: Supine, head supported on a pillow.

Therapist: Standing at the patient's head facing the shoulders.

Palpate: With both hands, grip the cranium in a palmar grip with the fingers directed caudally. With the fingertips of the index and long fingers, palpate the lateral aspect of the spinous process of the C2 vertebra bilaterally.

Localization: From a *neutral* position (not flexed or extended) rotate the atlanto–axial joints to the physiological limit by rotating the head until motion of the spinous process of the C2 vertebra is perceived. The limit of A/A rotation has been reached.

Mobilization: From this position, instruct the patient to turn the eyes to the desired direction of rotation, thus recruiting the appropriate rotator muscles of the A/A joints. This isometric contraction is held for 3–5 seconds following which the patient is instructed to completely relax. The new rotation barrier is localized. The mobilization is repeated 3 times.

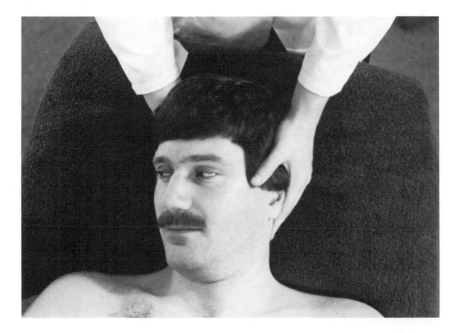

Notes:

_____

_____

_____

_____

_____

_____

_____

_____

_____

_____

_____

_____

_____

_____

_____

_____

_____

_____

_____

_____

_____

Midcervical Region

C2–3 to C6–7

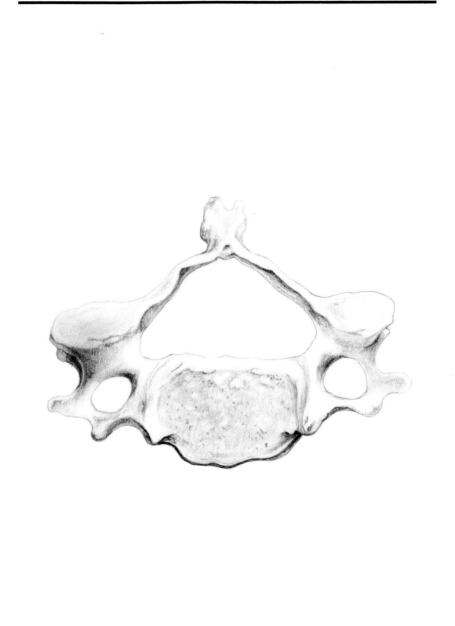

Midcervical Region — C2–3 to C6–7

1. POSITIONAL TESTS

Patient: Supine, head supported on a pillow.

Therapist: Standing at the patient's head facing the shoulders.

Palpate: With the index finger, palpate the lamina and the inferior articular process of the C2 vertebra bilaterally. The rest of the hand supports the cervical spine and the cranium.

Test: a) Hyperflexion: flex the joint complex and assess the position of the C2 vertebra relative to C3 by noting which lamina and inferior articular process is the most dorsal. A dorsal right inferior articular process of the C2 vertebra relative to C3 is indicative of a right rotated position of the C2-3 joint complex in hyperflexion.

b) Hyperextension: extend the joint complex and assess the position of the C2 vertebra relative to C3 by noting which lamina and inferior articular process is the most dorsal. A dorsal right inferior articular process of the C2 vertebra relative to C3 is indicative of a right rotated position of the C2-3 joint complex in hyperextension.

Repeat these tests for each segment.

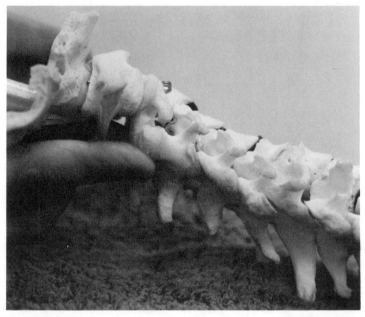

Notes:

_____

_____

_____

_____

_____

_____

_____

_____

_____

_____

_____

_____

_____

_____

_____

_____

_____

_____

_____

_____

_____

_____

2. MOBILITY TESTS — Specific Articular Mobility

a) Lateral Translation Mobility Test

Patient: Supine, head supported on a pillow.

Therapist: Standing at the patient's head facing the shoulders.

Palpate: With the tips of the index and long fingers, palpate the inferior articular process of the C2 vertebra bilaterally. The rest of the hand supports the cranium.

Test: a) Hyperflexion: flex the cervical spine. From this position, laterally translate (shear not sideflex) the C2-3 joint complex to the left and then to the right. Note the quantity and quality of motion.

b) Hyperextension: extend the cervical spine. From this position, laterally translate (shear not sideflex) the C2-3 joint complex to the left and then to the right. Note the quantity and quality of motion.

Repeat these tests for each segment.

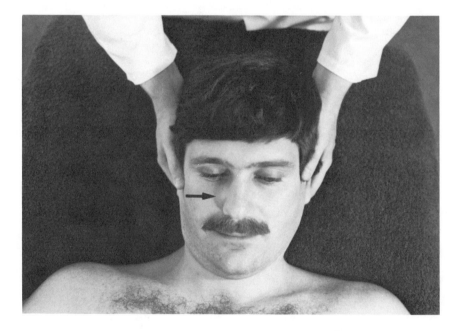

Notes:

_____

_____

_____

_____

_____

_____

_____

_____

_____

_____

_____

_____

_____

_____

_____

_____

_____

_____

_____

_____

_____

_____

_____

2. MOBILITY TESTS — Specific Articular Mobility
b) Passive Physiological Mobility Tests
1. Flexion/Extension

Patient: Supine, head supported on a pillow.

Therapist: Standing at the patient's head facing the shoulders.

Palpate: With the index and long fingers, palpate the inferior articular process of the C2 vertebra bilaterally. The rest of the hand supports the cranium.

Test: Flex/extend the C2–3 joint complex about the appropriate coronal axis. Note the quantity and quality of motion.

Repeat this test for each segment.

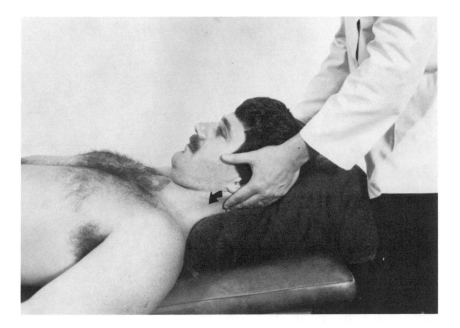

Notes:

_____

_____

_____

_____

_____

_____

_____

_____

_____

_____

_____

_____

_____

_____

_____

_____

_____

_____

_____

_____

_____

2. **MOBILITY TESTS — Specific Articular Mobility**
b) Passive Physiological Mobility Tests
2. Flexion/Sideflexion/Rotation

Patient: Supine, head supported on a pillow.

Therapist: Standing at the patient's head facing the shoulders.

Palpate: With the tips of the index and long fingers, palpate the inferior articular process of the C2 vertebra bilaterally. The rest of the hand supports the cranium.

Test: Flex the joint complex about the appropriate coronal axis. From this position, sideflex and rotate the C2–3 joint complex to the right and then to the left. Note the quantity and quality of motion.

Repeat this test for each segment.

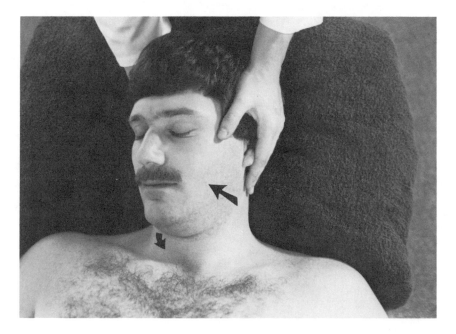

Notes:

_____

_____

_____

_____

_____

_____

_____

_____

_____

_____

_____

_____

_____

_____

_____

_____

_____

_____

_____

_____

_____

2. MOBILITY TESTS — Specific Articular Mobility

b) Passive Physiological Mobility Tests

3. Extension/Sideflexion/Rotation

Patient:	Supine, head supported on a pillow.
Therapist:	Standing at the patient's head facing the shoulders.
Palpate:	With the tips of the index and long fingers, palpate the inferior articular process of the C2 vertebra bilaterally.
Test:	Extend the joint complex about the appropriate coronal axis. From this position, sideflex and rotate the C2–3 joint complex to the right and then to the left. Note the quantity and quality of motion.
	Repeat this test for each segment.

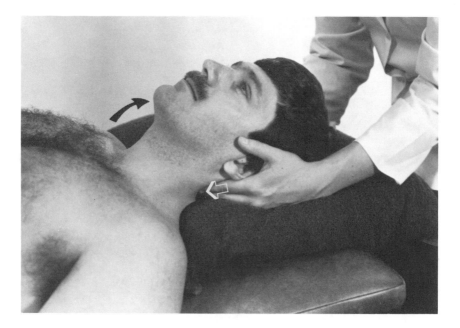

Notes:

_____

_____

_____

_____

_____

_____

_____

_____

_____

_____

_____

_____

_____

_____

_____

_____

_____

_____

_____

_____

_____

_____

3. STRESS TESTS

a) Ventral

Patient:	Supine, head supported on a pillow.
Therapist:	Standing at the patient's head facing the shoulders.
Palpate:	With the index fingers, palpate transversely the neural arch of the C2 vertebra. The rest of the hand supports the cranium.
Test:	Apply a slow, steady, ventral shear to the neural arch. This is restrained by the intervertebral disc and the associated longitudinal ligaments as well as the neural arch. Note the quantity and quality of motion.

Repeat this test for each segment.

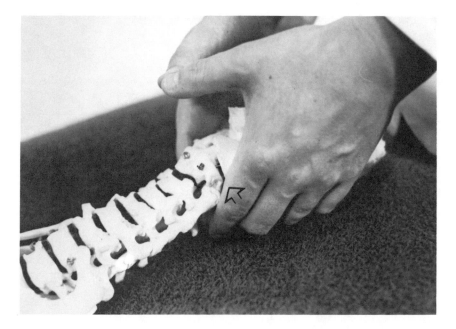

Notes:

_____

_____

_____

_____

_____

_____

_____

_____

_____

_____

_____

_____

_____

_____

_____

_____

_____

_____

_____

_____

_____

_____

3. STRESS TESTS

b) Dorsal

Patient:	Supine.
Therapist:	Standing at the patient's head facing the shoulders.
Palpate:	With the lateral aspect of the MCP joint of the index finger, palpate transversely the neural arch of the C3 vertebra. The ulnar border of this hand rests on the table. With an open pinch grip of the other hand, palpate the C2 vertebra.
Test:	Dorsally shear the C2 vertebra on C3. Note the quantity and quality of motion.

Repeat this test for each segment.

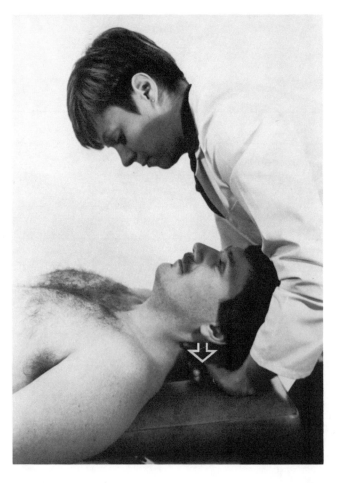

Notes:

_____

_____

_____

_____

_____

_____

_____

_____

_____

_____

_____

_____

_____

_____

_____

_____

_____

_____

_____

_____

_____

_____

_____

_____

3. STRESS TESTS

c) Lateral

Patient: Supine, head supported on a pillow.

Therapist: Standing at the patient's head facing the shoulders.

Palpate: With the lateral aspect of the MCP joint of the right index finger, palpate the right transverse process of the C2 vertebra. With the lateral aspect of the MCP joint of the left index finger, palpate the left transverse process of the C3 vertebra.

Test: Fix C3 and shear C2 transversely to the left. Switch hands and shear C2 to the right. This motion is primarily restrained by the uncinate processes of the caudal vertebral body. Note the quantity and quality of motion.

Repeat this test for each segment.

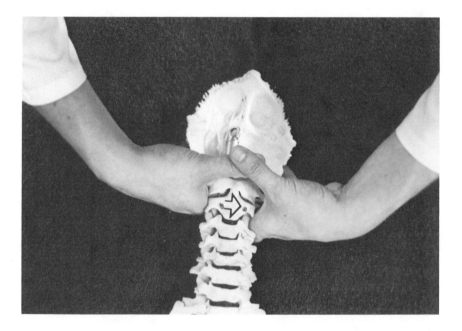

Notes:

_____

_____

_____

_____

_____

_____

_____

_____

_____

_____

_____

_____

_____

_____

_____

_____

_____

_____

_____

_____

_____

1. PASSIVE ARTICULAR MOBILIZATION

a) Specific Traction

Patient: Sitting, spine supported against the chair.

Therapist: Standing at the patient's side.

Palpate: With an open pinch grip of the dorsal hand, palpate the caudal vertebra of the joint complex. The rest of this hand supports the lower cervical spine. The medial border of the 5th digit of the ventral hand is applied to the lamina and inferior articular process of the cranial vertebra. The rest of this hand supports the cranium and the upper cervical spine.

Localization: Localization is achieved by a facet lock of the cranial chain of bones. Incongruent sideflexion and rotation are used to lock the upper cervical units. Example: the *To barrier* cervical spine is sideflexed *away from* and rotated *towards* the therapist just to the level above that being treated. Care must be taken to ensure that the joint being treated remains in *neutral.*

Mobilization: Fix the caudal vertebra and traction the joint complex by straightening the knees. No specific hand motion is required.

No finger tip locking — lumbrical lock!

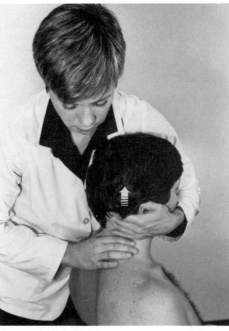

MIDCERVICAL REGION   TREATMENT

Notes:

Remember to traction at angle of facet — more C6 on C5 ∴ hand pushing down at an angle to distract

For a disc, head moves forwards and upwards, lumbrical grip for lower neck & grade 1 is breathing
heel on rest of neck
to fix

Knees pointing out,
pts. head into therapist shldr
elbow of therapist at chin,
P.T. = one foot behind & along side
always S.B. away

MIDCERVICAL REGION   TREATMENT

1. PASSIVE ARTICULAR MOBILIZATION

b) Flexion/Sideflexion/Rotation

Rotation is conjoined with ipsilateral sideflexion in this region of the spine and a combined technique is the most effective. Pure rotation as a treatment technique is detrimental to the health of the joint since this motion is unphysiological.

Patient: Sitting, spine supported against the chair.

Therapist: Standing at the patient's side.

Palpate: With an open pinch grip of the dorsal hand, palpate the caudal vertebra of the joint complex. The rest of this hand supports the lower cervical spine. The medial border of the 5th digit of the ventral hand is applied to the lamina and inferior articular process of the cranial vertebra. The rest of this hand supports the cranium and the upper cervical spine.

Localization: Localization is achieved by a facet lock of the cranial chain of bones. Incongruent sideflexion and rotation are used to lock the upper cervical units. Example: the cervical spine is sideflexed *away from* and rotated *towards* the therapist just to the level above that being treated. Care must be taken to ensure that the joint being treated remains in *neutral*.

to berrier

Mobilization: With the 5th digit of the ventral hand, flex, sideflex, and ipsilaterally rotate the joint complex. The dorsal hand fixes the caudal vertebra. The direction of pull is cranial and medial.

This technique can also be done with the patient supine.

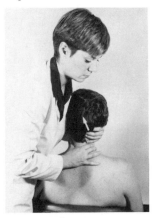

Notes:

with loss of flexion

lock to level by flexing, S.B. &
rotate to opposite side

Need to treat from opposite side
of facet dysfunction.

Mobilize from knee
Little finger over lamina.
Stabilizing arm - elbow into side
(will move - a counterforce)

Lock the Same as Specific traction

MIDCERVICAL REGION   TREATMENT

1. PASSIVE ARTICULAR MOBILIZATION
c) Extension/Sideflexion/Rotation

Rotation is conjoined with ipsilateral sideflexion in this region of the spine and a combined technique is the most effective. Pure rotation as a treatment technique is detrimental to the health of the joint since this motion is unphysiological.

Patient: Sitting, spine supported against the chair.

Therapist: Standing at the patient's side.

Palpate: With an open pinch grip of the dorsal hand, palpate the caudal vertebra of the joint complex. The rest of this hand supports the lower cervical spine. The medial border of the 5th digit of the ventral hand is applied to the lamina and inferior articular process of the cranial vertebra. The rest of this hand supports the cranium and the upper cervical spine.

Localization: Localization is achieved by a facet lock of the cranial chain of bones. Incongruent sideflexion and rotation are used to lock the upper cervical units. Example: the cervical spine is sideflexed *away from* and rotated *towards* the therapist just to the level above that being treated. Care must be taken to ensure that the joint being treated remains in *neutral*.

Mobilization: With the 5th digit of the ventral hand, extend, side-flex, and ipsilaterally rotate the joint complex. The dorsal hand fixes the caudal vertebra. The direction of push is caudal and medial.

This technique can also be done with the patient supine.

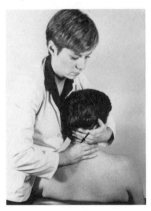

Notes:

Specific Traction position

Fix head & rotate inferior segment

1. PASSIVE ARTICULAR MOBILIZATION

d) General Traction

Patient: Supine, head supported on a pillow.

Therapist: Standing at the patient's head facing the shoulders.

Palpate: With one hand, support the occiput. With the other hand, cradle the mandible.

Localization: The degree of cervical flexion determines the level of localization.

Mobilization: Apply the traction force by slowly leaning backwards. The hand supporting the mandible is used only to guide the movement thus avoiding compression of the temporomandibular joints.

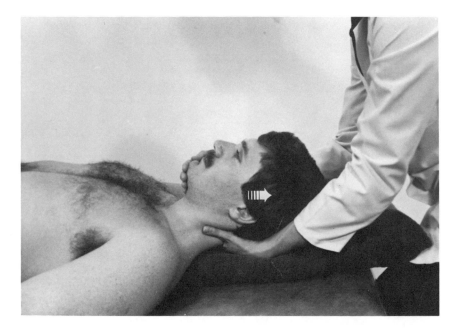

Notes:

1. PASSIVE ARTICULAR MOBILIZATION

e) Posteroanterior Pressures (P/A's)

Patient: Prone, head in a sagittal plane.

Therapist: Standing at the patient's head facing the shoulders.

Palpate: The pads of the thumbs are used to transmit the force to the joint.

Mobilization: Posteroanterior pressures can be applied to the spinous process or unilaterally to the articular pillar. The depth and direction of the pressure is dictated by the health and the anatomy of the joint being treated. The mobilization force is applied through straight arms.

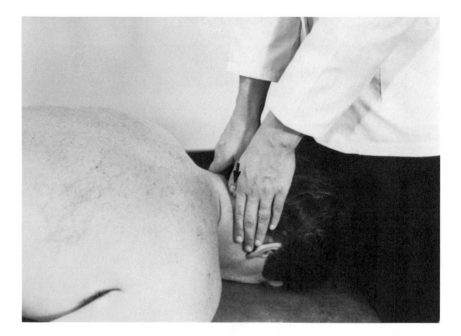

Notes:

_____

_____

_____

_____

_____

_____

_____

_____

_____

_____

_____

_____

_____

_____

_____

_____

_____

_____

_____

_____

_____

_____

2. ACTIVE MOBILIZATION

a) Flexion/Sideflexion/Rotation

Patient: Sitting, spine supported against the chair.

Therapist: Standing at the patient's side.

Palpate: With an open pinch grip of the dorsal hand, palpate the caudal vertebra of the joint complex. The rest of this hand supports the lower cervical spine. The medial border of the 5th digit of the ventral hand is applied to the lamina and inferior articular process of the cranial vertebra. The rest of this hand supports the cranium and the upper cervical spine.

Localization: The motion barrier is localized by flexing, sideflexing and ipsilaterally rotating the joint complex to the physiological limit. It is extremely important that the axes about which these motions are induced are segmentally accurate.

Mobilization: From this position, the patient is instructed to hold the head still while the therapist applies a gentle resistance to the cranium (arrow). This isometric contraction may be either towards or away from the desired direction of mobilization and is held for 3–5 seconds following which the patient is instructed to completely relax. The new flexion/sideflexion/rotation barrier is localized. The mobilization is repeated 3 times.

This technique can also be done with the patient supine.

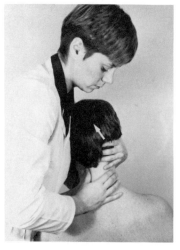

Notes:

_____

_____

_____

_____

_____

_____

_____

_____

_____

_____

_____

_____

_____

_____

_____

_____

_____

_____

_____

_____

2. ACTIVE MOBILIZATION

b) Extension/Sideflexion/Rotation

Patient: Sitting, spine supported against the chair.

Therapist: Standing at the patient's side.

Palpate: With an open pinch grip of the dorsal hand, palpate the caudal vertebra of the joint complex. The rest of this hand supports the lower cervical spine. The medial border of the 5th digit of the ventral hand is applied to the lamina and inferior articular process of the cranial vertebra. The rest of this hand supports the cranium and the upper cervical spine.

Localization: The motion barrier is localized by extending, sideflexing and ipsilaterally rotating the joint complex to the physiological limit. It is extremely important that the axes about which these motions are induced are segmentally accurate.

Mobilization: From this position, the patient is instructed to hold the head still while the therapist applies a gentle resistance to the cranium (arrow). This isometric contraction may be either towards or away from the desired direction of mobilization and is held for 3–5 seconds following which the patient is instructed to completely relax. The new extension/sideflexion/rotation barrier is localized. The mobilization is repeated 3 times.

This technique can also be done with the patient supine.

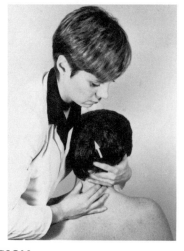

Notes:

_____

_____

_____

_____

_____

_____

_____

_____

_____

_____

_____

_____

_____

_____

_____

_____

_____

_____

_____

_____

_____

_____

Cervicothoracic Region

C7–T1 to T2–3, Ribs 1 and 2

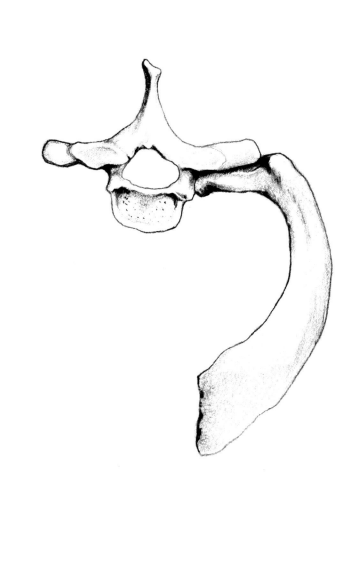

Cervicothoracic Region — C7–T1 to T2–3, Ribs 1 and 2

A. SPINAL

1. POSITIONAL TESTS

Patient: Sitting, spine supported against the chair.

Therapist: Standing behind the patient.

Palpate: With the thumbs, palpate the transverse processes of the C7 vertebra.

Test: a) Hyperflexion: flex the joint complex and assess the position of the C7 vertebra relative to T1 by noting which transverse process is the most dorsal. A dorsal left transverse process of C7 relative to T1 is indicative of a left rotated position of the C7–T1 joint complex in hyperflexion.

b) Hyperextension: extend the joint complex and assess the position of the C7 vertebra relative to T1 by noting which transverse process is the most dorsal. A dorsal left transverse process of C7 relative to T1 is indicative of a left rotated position of the C7–T1 joint complex in hyperextension.

Repeat these tests for each segment.

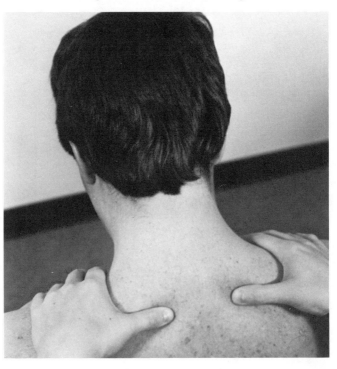

Notes:

_____

_____

_____

_____

_____

_____

_____

_____

_____

_____

_____

_____

_____

_____

_____

_____

_____

_____

_____

_____

_____

A. **SPINAL**
2. **MOBILITY TESTS — Specific Articular Mobility**
   a) Active Physiological Mobility Tests

Patient:	Sitting, spine supported against the chair.
	1. Method A — Dorsal
Therapist:	Standing behind the patient.
Palpate:	With the thumbs, palpate the transverse processes of the C7 vertebra.
	2. Method B — Ventral
Therapist:	Standing in front of the patient.
Palpate:	With the index fingers or thumbs, palpate the cranial aspect of the 2nd rib at the manubriocostal junction bilaterally.
Test:	a) Instruct the patient to flex the head forward and note the relative displacement of the transverse processes/ribs.
	b) Instruct the patient to extend the head modifying the motion such that the segment being examined is in fact extending since habitual extension of the head on the thorax induces cervicothoracic flexion. Note the relative displacement of the transverse processes/ribs.
	Asymmetry *may* be indicative of dysfunction. Repeat these tests for each segment.

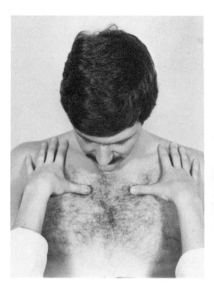 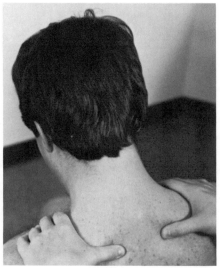

Notes:

_____

_____

_____

_____

_____

_____

_____

_____

_____

_____

_____

_____

_____

_____

_____

_____

_____

_____

_____

_____

A. **SPINAL**

2. **MOBILITY TESTS — Specific Articular Mobility**

   b) Passive Physiological Mobility Tests

      1. Flexion/Extension

Patient:	Sitting, spine supported against the chair.
Therapist:	Standing at the patient's side.
Palpate:	With the index finger of the dorsal hand, palpate the interspinous space of the C7–T1 segment. The medial border of the 5th digit of the ventral hand is applied to the lamina and inferior articular process of the C7 vertebra. The rest of this hand supports the cervical spine and the arm cradles the cranium.
Test:	Passively flex/extend the joint complex about the appropriate coronal axis and note the quantity and quality of motion.

                   Repeat this test for each segment.

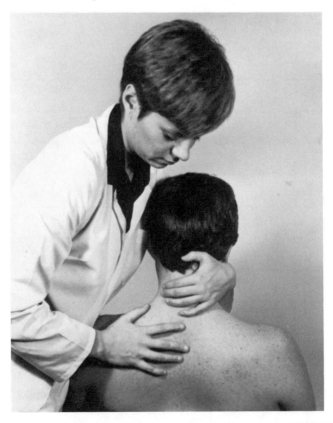

Notes:

_____

_____

_____

_____

_____

_____

_____

_____

_____

_____

_____

_____

_____

_____

_____

_____

_____

_____

_____

_____

_____

A. **SPINAL**
2. **MOBILITY TESTS — Specific Articular Mobility**
   b) Passive Physiological Mobility Tests
      2. Sideflexion/Rotation

Patient:	Sitting, spine supported against the chair.
Therapist:	Standing at the patient's side.
Palpate:	With the index finger of the dorsal hand, palpate the interspinous space of the C7–T1 segment. The medial border of the 5th digit of the ventral hand is applied to the lamina and inferior articular process of the C7 vertebra. The rest of this hand supports the cervical spine and the arm cradles the cranium.
Test:	With the joint complex in a neutral position:

a) Sideflexion — Passively sideflex the joint complex about the appropriate sagittal axis. Note the quantity and quality of motion.

b) Rotation — Passively rotate the joint complex about the appropriate vertical axis. Note the quantity and quality of motion.

c) Combined Sideflexion/Rotation — Passively sideflex/rotate the joint complex about the appropriate oblique axis. Repeat the test in hyperflexion and hyperextension. Note the quantity and quality of motion.

Repeat these tests for each segment.

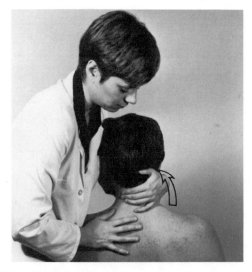

Notes:

_____

_____

_____

_____

_____

_____

_____

_____

_____

_____

_____

_____

_____

_____

_____

_____

_____

_____

_____

_____

B. COSTAL

1. POSITIONAL TESTS

Patient:	Sitting, spine supported against the chair.
	a) Method A — Dorsal
Therapist:	Standing behind the patient.
Palpate:	With the thumbs, palpate the rib just lateral to the tubercle and medial to the angle bilaterally.
	b) Method B — Ventral
Therapist:	Standing in front of the patient.
Palpate:	1st Rib — With the index fingers or thumbs, palpate the ventral aspect of the first rib at the manubriocostal junction bilaterally.
	2nd Rib — With the index fingers or thumbs, palpate the ventral and then the cranial aspect of the second rib at the manubriocostal junction bilaterally.
Test:	Note the craniocaudal, ventrodorsal relationship of the two ribs (L/R).

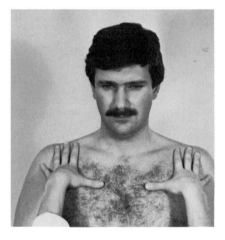 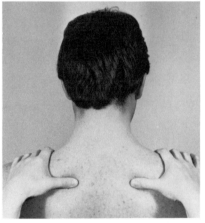

Notes:

_____

_____

_____

_____

_____

_____

_____

_____

_____

_____

_____

_____

_____

_____

_____

_____

_____

_____

_____

_____

_____

B. **COSTAL**

2. **MOBILITY TESTS — Specific Articular Mobility**

    a) Active Physiological Mobility Tests

        1. Method A — Dorsal

Patient:	Sitting, spine supported against the chair.
Therapist:	Standing behind the patient.
Palpate:	With the thumbs, palpate the ribs just lateral to the tubercle and medial to the angle.
Test:	a) Instruct the patient to inspire fully and note the quantity and quality of motion. Any restriction or deviant movement pattern *may* be indicative of dysfunction.
	b) Instruct the patient to expire fully and note the quantity and quality of motion. Any restriction or deviant movement pattern *may* be indicative of dysfunction.

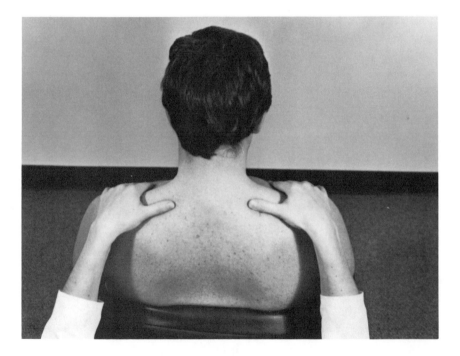

Notes:

_____

_____

_____

_____

_____

_____

_____

_____

_____

_____

_____

_____

_____

_____

_____

_____

_____

_____

_____

_____

B. **COSTAL**

2. **MOBILITY TESTS — Specific Articular Mobility**

  a) Active Physiological Mobility Tests

    2. Method B — Ventral

Patient:	Sitting, spine supported against the chair.
Therapist:	Standing in front of the patient.
Palpate:	1st Rib — with the index fingers or thumbs, palpate the ventral aspect of the first rib at the manubriocostal junction bilaterally.
	2nd Rib — with the index fingers or thumbs, palpate the cranial aspect of the second rib at the manubriocostal junction bilaterally.
Test:	a) Instruct the patient to inspire fully and note the quantity and quality of motion. Any restriction or deviant movement pattern *may* be indicative of dysfunction.
	b) Instruct the patient to expire fully and note the quantity and quality of motion. Any restriction or deviant movement pattern *may* be indicative of dysfunction.

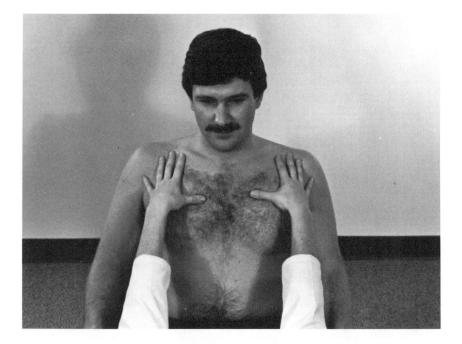

Notes:

_____

_____

_____

_____

_____

_____

_____

_____

_____

_____

_____

_____

_____

_____

_____

_____

_____

_____

_____

_____

_____

_____

B. **COSTAL**

2. **MOBILITY TESTS — Specific Articular Mobility**

   b) Passive Accessory Mobility Test

      Patient: Sitting, spine supported against the chair.

      Therapist: Standing behind the patient.

      Palpate: With the thumb, palpate the rib just lateral to the tubercle and medial to the angle.

      Test: Apply a posteroanterior pressure along the line of the neck of the rib. This direction is determined by the angle formed between the neck of the rib and the coronal plane. Note the quantity and quality of motion.

                  Repeat this test for each rib.

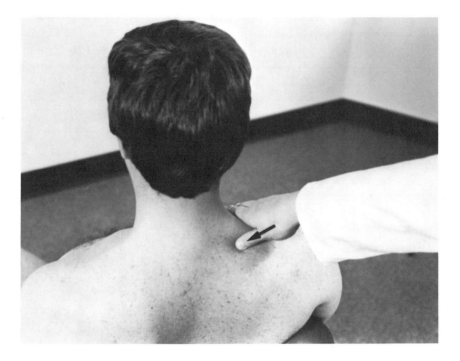

Notes:

_____

_____

_____

_____

_____

_____

_____

_____

_____

_____

_____

_____

_____

_____

_____

_____

_____

_____

_____

_____

A. SPINAL

1. PASSIVE ARTICULAR MOBILIZATION

a) Extension

Patient: Supine, head supported by the therapist.

Therapist: Standing at the patient's head facing the shoulders.

Palpate: With the lateral aspect of the MCP joint of the index finger, palpate transversely the caudal vertebra of the joint complex. The opposite hand cups the cervical spine and the cranium.

Mobilization: Dorsally glide the joint complex by allowing the cervical spine and the cranium to descend on the fixed caudal vertebra.

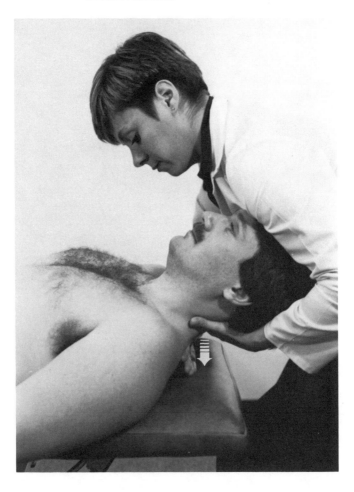

Notes:

_____

_____

_____

_____

_____

_____

_____

_____

_____

_____

_____

_____

_____

_____

_____

_____

_____

_____

_____

A. **SPINAL**

1. **PASSIVE ARTICULAR MOBILIZATION**

   b) Rotation/Sideflexion

   Rotation is not a pure movement in this region; it is conjoined with a small degree of sideflexion. The direction of 'ease of motion' must be located and the mobilization technique applied in this plane.

   Patient: Sitting, spine supported against the chair.

   Therapist: Standing at the patient's side.

   Palpate: With the dorsal hand, fix the caudal vertebra of the joint complex by applying pressure to the spinous process on the contralateral side with the thumb. The medial border of the 4th or 5th digit of the ventral hand is applied to the lamina and inferior articular process, or hooked around the spinous process, of the cranial vertebra. The rest of this hand supports the cervical spine while the arm cradles the cranium.

   Mobilization: The direction of 'ease of motion' for rotation/sideflexion is located and the mobilization technique applied in this plane. This can be an extremely effective technique for the restoration of axial extension if combined with a dorsal glide.

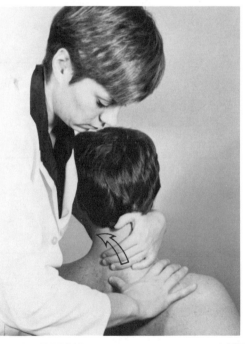

Notes:

_____

_____

_____

_____

_____

_____

_____

_____

_____

_____

_____

_____

_____

_____

_____

_____

_____

_____

_____

_____

A. SPINAL
1. PASSIVE ARTICULAR MOBILIZATION
c) Traction

Patient: Sitting or standing, hands placed behind the neck with the fingers interlaced.

Therapist: Standing behind the patient.

Palpate: Wind both arms under the patient's axillae to place the hands on the back of the neck. With the thumbs directed caudally, interlace the fingers and hook the thumbs underneath the spinous process of the cranial vertebra of the joint complex being treated. Gently grip the thorax under the axillae with the inner arms.

Mobilization: Instruct the patient to look forward in order to release the ligamentum nuchae. Rock the patient backwards, allowing gravity to traction the joint complex.

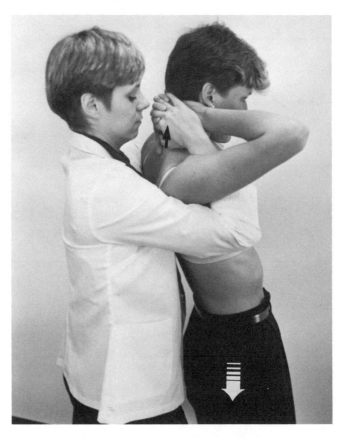

Notes:

_____

_____

_____

_____

_____

_____

_____

_____

_____

_____

_____

_____

_____

_____

_____

_____

_____

_____

_____

_____

_____

_____

A. SPINAL
2. ACTIVE MOBILIZATION
a) Extension

Patient: Supine, head supported by the therapist.

Therapist: Standing at the patient's head facing the shoulders.

Palpate: With the lateral aspect of the MCP joint of the index finger, palpate transversely the caudal vertebra of the joint complex. The opposite hand cups the cervical spine and the cranium.

Localization: The motion barrier is localized by gently gliding the joint complex dorsally to the limit.

Mobilization: From this position, the patient is instructed to hold the head still while the therapist minimally releases the support of the cranial hand. This isometric contraction is held for 3–5 seconds. Full support is reapplied and the patient is instructed to completely relax. The new dorsal glide barrier is localized. The mobilization is repeated 3 times.

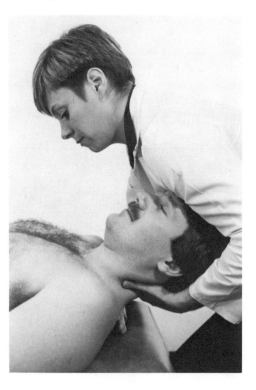

Notes:

_____

_____

_____

_____

_____

_____

_____

_____

_____

_____

_____

_____

_____

_____

_____

_____

_____

_____

_____

_____

_____

_____

A. **SPINAL**

2. **ACTIVE MOBILIZATION**

   b) Flexion/Sideflexion/Rotation

   Patient: Sitting, spine supported against the chair.

   Therapist: Standing at the patient's side.

   Palpate: With the index finger of the dorsal hand, palpate the interspinous space of the segment. The ventral hand cups the cervical spine while the arm cradles the cranium.

   Localization: The motion barrier is localized by flexing, sideflexing and rotating the joint complex to the physiological limit. Accurate localization is essential for the success of this technique.

   Mobilization: From this position, the patient is instructed to hold the head still while the therapist applies a minimal force towards the midline (arrow). This isometric contraction is held for 3–5 seconds following which the patient is instructed to completely relax. The new flexion/sideflexion/rotation barrier is localized. The mobilization is repeated 3 times.

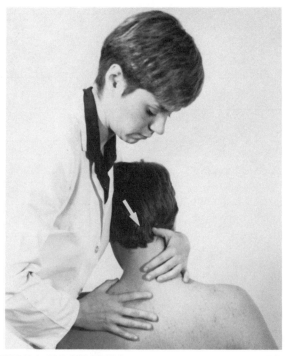

Notes:

_____

_____

_____

_____

_____

_____

_____

_____

_____

_____

_____

_____

_____

_____

_____

_____

_____

_____

_____

_____

_____

_____

_____

A. **SPINAL**

2. **ACTIVE MOBILIZATION**

   c) Extension/Sideflexion/Rotation

     Patient: Sitting, spine supported against the chair.

     Therapist: Standing at the patient's side.

     Palpate: With the index finger of the dorsal hand, palpate the interspinous space of the segment. The ventral hand cups the cervical spine while the arm cradles the cranium.

     Localization: The motion barrier is localized by extending, sideflexing and rotating the joint complex to the physiological limit. Accurate localization is essential for the success of this technique.

     Mobilization: From this position, the patient is instructed to hold the head still while the therapist applies a minimal force towards the midline (arrow). This isometric contraction is held for 3–5 seconds following which the patient is instructed to completely relax. The new extension/sideflexion/rotation barrier is localized.

       The mobilization is repeated 3 times.

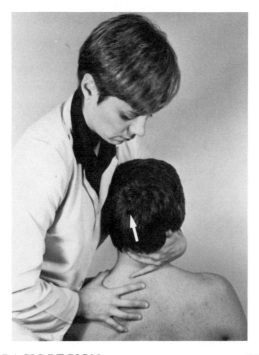

Notes:

_____

_____

_____

_____

_____

_____

_____

_____

_____

_____

_____

_____

_____

_____

_____

_____

_____

_____

_____

_____

_____

_____

B. COSTAL
1. PASSIVE ARTICULAR MOBILIZATION

Patient: Supine, head supported on a pillow.

Therapist: Standing at the patient's head facing the shoulders.

Palpate: With the lateral aspect of the MCP joint of the index finger, palpate the craniodorsal aspect of the rib just lateral to the tubercle. The cranium and the cervical spine are supported by a palmar grip of the opposite hand.

Localization: Lock the cervicothoracic spine by sideflexing the neck towards the rib being treated about a sagittal axis through the manubrium, and then rotating the neck away from that rib. This localization is done with the hand supporting the cranium and the cervical spine.

Mobilization: Apply a caudal/ventral pressure along the line of the neck of the rib.

Addendum: The ipsilateral scalene muscles may be inhibited by recruitment of those on the contralateral side. The patient is instructed to hold the head still while the therapist attempts to increase the sideflexion component of the localization. The rib can be further mobilized in a caudal/ventral direction during this inhibition.

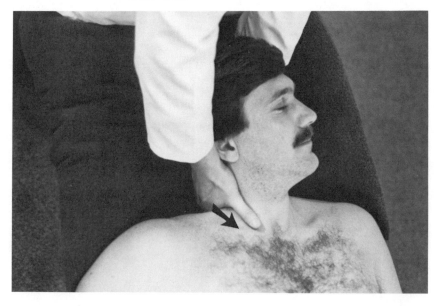

Notes:

_____

_____

_____

_____

_____

_____

_____

_____

_____

_____

_____

_____

_____

_____

_____

_____

_____

_____

_____

_____

_____

Thoracic Region
T3–4 to T10–11, Ribs 3–12

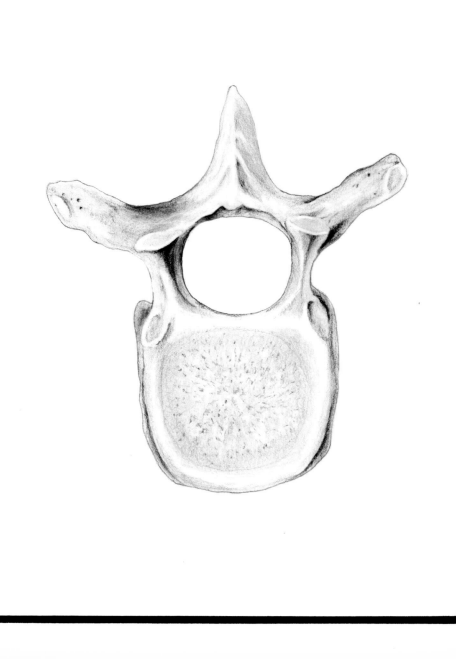

Thoracic Region — T3–4 to T10–11, Ribs 3–12

A. SPINAL

1. POSITIONAL TESTS

a) Hyperflexion

Patient:	Sitting, feet supported, thoracic spine fully flexed.
Therapist:	Standing behind the patient.
Palpate:	With the thumbs, palpate the transverse processes of the T3 vertebra.
Test:	Assess the position of the T3 vertebra relative to T4 by noting which transverse process is the most dorsal. A dorsal left transverse process of T3 relative to T4 is indicative of a left rotated position of the T3-4 joint complex in hyperflexion.

Repeat this test for each segment.

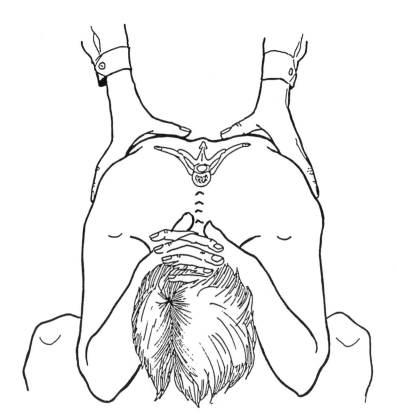

Notes:

_____

_____

_____

_____

_____

_____

_____

_____

_____

_____

_____

_____

_____

_____

_____

_____

_____

_____

_____

_____

_____

_____

A. **SPINAL**

1. **POSITIONAL TESTS**

b) Hyperextension

Patient:	Prone, thoracic spine fully extended, chin resting in the hands.
Therapist:	Standing at the patient's side.
Palpate:	With the thumbs, palpate the transverse processes of the T3 vertebra.
Test:	Assess the position of the T3 vertebra relative to T4 by noting which transverse process is the most dorsal. A dorsal left transverse process of T3 relative to T4 is indicative of a left rotated position of the T3–4 joint complex in hyperextension.

Repeat this test for each segment.

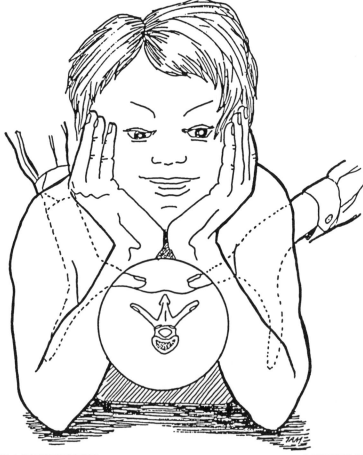

Notes:

A. SPINAL

2. MOBILITY TESTS — Specific Articular Mobility

a) Active Physiological Mobility Tests

Patient: Sitting, feet supported.

Therapist: Standing behind the patient.

Palpate: With the thumbs, palpate the transverse processes of the T3 vertebra.

Test: a) Instruct the patient to flex the spine forward and note the cranial/ventral displacement of the transverse processes. Asymmetry *may* be indicative of dysfunction.

b) Instruct the patient to extend the spine and note the caudal displacement of the transverse processes. Asymmetry *may* be indicative of dysfunction.

Repeat these tests for each segment.

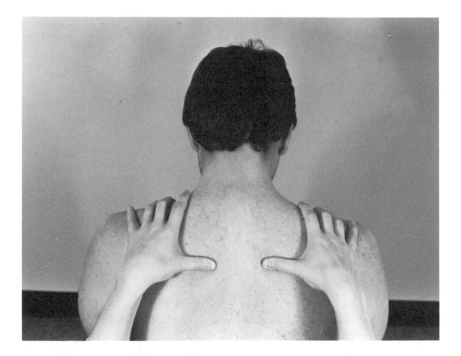

Notes:

_____

_____

_____

_____

_____

_____

_____

_____

_____

_____

_____

_____

_____

_____

_____

_____

_____

_____

_____

_____

_____

_____

A. SPINAL
2. MOBILITY TESTS — Specific Articular Mobility
b) Passive Physiological Mobility Tests
1. Flexion/Extension

Patient: Sitting, feet supported, arms crossed to opposite shoulders.

Therapist: Standing at the patient's side.

Palpate: With the index finger of the dorsal hand, palpate the interspinous space of the segment. For the upper thoracic region, the ventral hand is wound through the patient's crossed arms to rest on the contralateral shoulder. For the lower joints, the ventral hand is placed on the contralateral scapula, the arm resting against the patient's chest.

Test: Passively flex/extend the joint complex about the appropriate coronal axis and note the quantity and quality of motion.

Repeat this test for each segment.

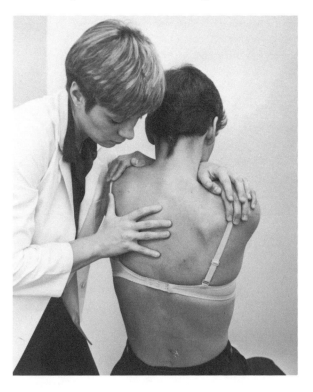

Notes:

_____

_____

_____

_____

_____

_____

_____

_____

_____

_____

_____

_____

_____

_____

_____

_____

_____

_____

_____

_____

_____

A. **SPINAL**

2. **MOBILITY TESTS — Specific Articular Mobility**

   b) Passive Physiological Mobility Tests

      2. Sideflexion/Rotation

Patient:	Sitting, feet supported, arms crossed to opposite shoulders.
Therapist:	Standing at the patient's side.
Palpate:	With the index finger of the dorsal hand, palpate the interspinous space of the segment. For the upper thoracic region, the ventral hand is wound through the patient's crossed arms to rest on the contralateral shoulder. For the lower joints, the ventral hand is placed on the contralateral scapula, the arm resting against the patient's chest.
Test:	With the joint complex in a neutral position:

a) Sideflexion — passively sideflex the joint complex about the appropriate sagittal axis and note the quantity and quality of motion.

b) Rotation — passively rotate the joint complex about the appropriate vertical axis and note the quantity and quality of motion.

c) Combined Sideflexion/Rotation — passively sideflex/rotate the joint complex about the appropriate oblique axis. Repeat the test in hyperflexion and then in hyperextension. Note the quantity and quality of motion.

Repeat these tests for each segment.

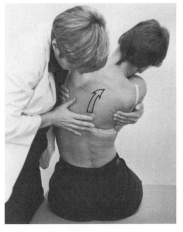

Notes:

_____

_____

_____

_____

_____

_____

_____

_____

_____

_____

_____

_____

_____

_____

_____

_____

_____

_____

_____

_____

_____

A. **SPINAL**

2. **MOBILITY TESTS — Specific Articular Mobility**

    c) Passive Accessory Mobility Tests

       1. Posteroanterior Pressures (P/A's)

       a) Hyperflexion

Patient:	Sitting, feet supported, thoracic spine flexed.
Therapist:	Standing behind the patient.
Palpate:	With the thumb, palpate the transverse process of the T3 vertebra.
Test:	Apply a posteroanterior pressure unilaterally to the transverse process of the T3 vertebra. Note the quantity and quality of motion.

               Repeat this test bilaterally for each segment.

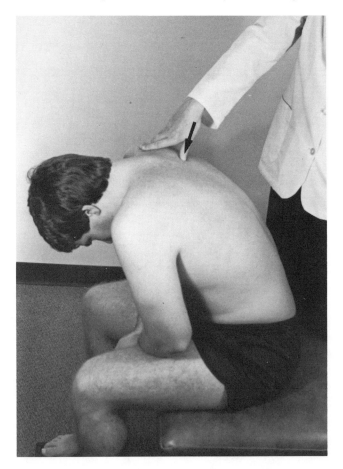

Notes:

_____

_____

_____

_____

_____

_____

_____

_____

_____

_____

_____

_____

_____

_____

_____

_____

_____

_____

_____

_____

_____

_____

A. **SPINAL**

2. **MOBILITY TESTS — Specific Articular Mobility**
    c) Passive Accessory Mobility Tests
        1. Posteroanterior Pressures (P/A's)
        b) Hyperextension

Patient:	Prone, thoracic spine fully extended, chin resting in the hands.
Therapist:	Standing at the patient's side.
Palpate:	With the thumbs, palpate the transverse processes of the T3 vertebra.
Test:	Apply a posteroanterior pressure unilaterally to the transverse processes of the T3 vertebra. Note the quantity and quality of motion.
	Repeat this test for each segment.

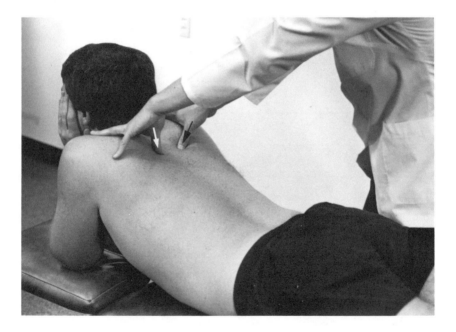

Notes:

_____

_____

_____

_____

_____

_____

_____

_____

_____

_____

_____

_____

_____

_____

_____

_____

_____

_____

_____

_____

_____

_____

B. COSTAL
1. POSITIONAL TESTS
a) Dorsal

Patient:	Prone.
Therapist:	Standing at the patient's side.
Palpate:	With the thumbs, palpate the ribs just lateral to the tubercle and medial to the angle.
Test:	Note the ventrodorsal relationship of the two ribs (L/R).

Repeat this test for each rib.

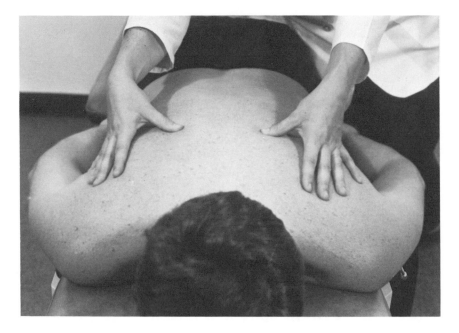

Notes:

_____

_____

_____

_____

_____

_____

_____

_____

_____

_____

_____

_____

_____

_____

_____

_____

_____

_____

_____

_____

B. COSTAL

1. POSITIONAL TESTS

  b) Ventral

Patient:	Supine.
Therapist:	Standing at the patient's head facing the shoulders.
Palpate:	With the index fingers or thumbs, palpate the ventral and then the cranial aspect of the two ribs (L/R) at the sternocostal junction.
Test:	Note the ventrodorsal/craniocaudal relationship of the two ribs (L/R).

Repeat this test for each rib.

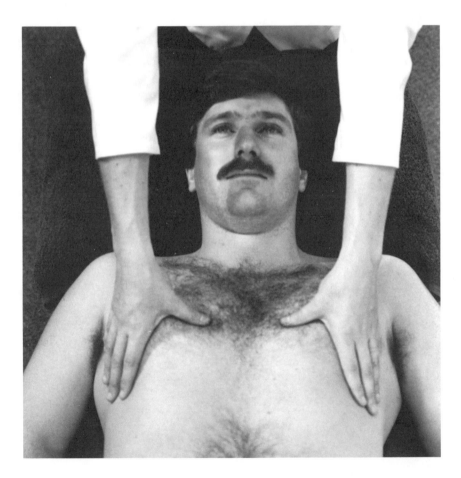

Notes:

B. **COSTAL**
1. **POSITIONAL TESTS**
    c) Lateral

        Patient: Supine.

        Therapist: Standing at the patient's side.

        Palpate: With the index fingers, palpate the lateral aspect of the two ribs (L/R) in the midaxillary line.

        Test: Note the craniocaudal, external rotation/internal rotation relationship of the two ribs (L/R).

                     Repeat this test for each rib.

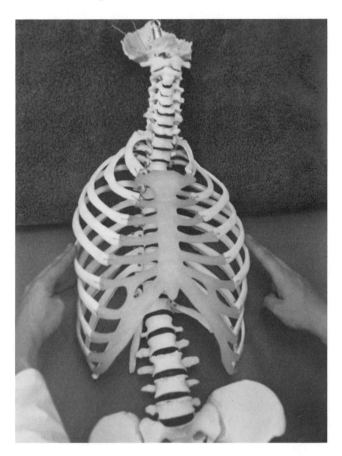

Notes:

_____

_____

_____

_____

_____

_____

_____

_____

_____

_____

_____

_____

_____

_____

_____

_____

_____

_____

_____

_____

_____

B. **COSTAL**

2. **MOBILITY TESTS — Specific Articular Mobility**

  a) Active Physiological Mobility Tests

    1. Method A — Dorsal

Patient: Prone.

Therapist: Standing beside the patient.

Palpate: With the thumbs, palpate the ribs just lateral to the tubercle and medial to the angle.

Test: a) Instruct the patient to inspire fully and note the quantity and quality of motion. Asymmetry *may* be indicative of dysfunction.

b) Instruct the patient to expire fully and note the quantity and quality of motion. Asymmetry *may* be indicative of dysfunction.

Repeat these tests for each rib.

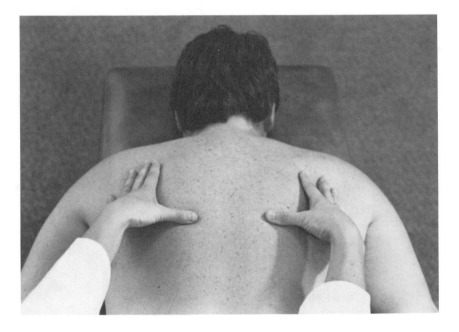

Notes:

_____

_____

_____

_____

_____

_____

_____

_____

_____

_____

_____

_____

_____

_____

_____

_____

_____

_____

_____

_____

_____

_____

B. **COSTAL**

2. **MOBILITY TESTS — Specific Articular Mobility**

   a) Active Physiological Mobility Tests

      2. Method B — Ventral

      Patient: Supine.

      Therapist: Standing at the patient's head facing the shoulders.

      Palpate: With the index fingers or thumbs, palpate the cranial aspect of the ribs at the sternocostal junction.

      Test: a) Instruct the patient to inspire fully and note the quantity and quality of motion. Asymmetry *may* be indicative of dysfunction.

      b) Instruct the patient to expire fully and note the quantity and quality of motion. Asymmetry *may* be indicative of dysfunction.

      Repeat these tests for each rib.

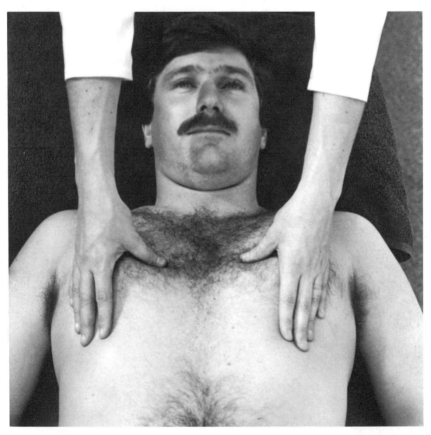

Notes:

_____

_____

_____

_____

_____

_____

_____

_____

_____

_____

_____

_____

_____

_____

_____

_____

_____

_____

_____

_____

B. **COSTAL**

2. **MOBILITY TESTS — Specific Articular Mobility**

   a) Active Physiological Mobility Tests

      3. Method C — Lateral

Patient:	Supine.
Therapist:	Standing at the patient's side.
Palpate:	With the index fingers, palpate the lateral aspect of the ribs in the midaxillary line.
Test:	a) Instruct the patient to inspire fully and note the quantity and quality of motion. Asymmetry *may* be indicative of dysfunction.
	b) Instruct the patient to expire fully and note the quantity and quality of motion. Asymmetry *may* be indicative of dysfunction.

              Repeat these tests for each rib.

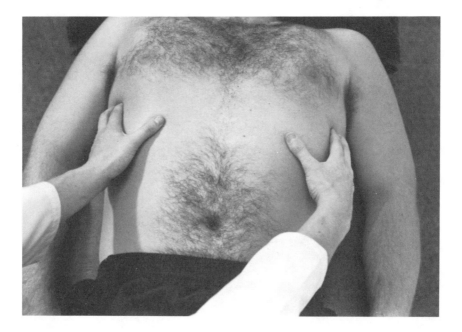

Notes:

_____

_____

_____

_____

_____

_____

_____

_____

_____

_____

_____

_____

_____

_____

_____

_____

_____

_____

_____

_____

B. COSTAL

2. MOBILITY TESTS — Specific Articular Mobility

b) Passive Accessory Mobility Test

Patient:	Prone.
Therapist:	Standing at the patient's side.
Palpate:	With the thumbs, palpate the rib just lateral to the tubercle and medial to the angle.
Test:	Apply a posteroanterior pressure along the line of the neck of the rib. This direction is determined by the angle formed between the neck of the rib and the coronal plane. Note the quantity and quality of motion.

Repeat this test for each rib.

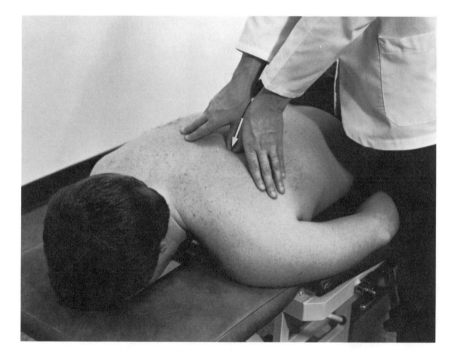

Notes:

A. SPINAL
1. PASSIVE ARTICULAR MOBILIZATION
a) Flexion

Patient: Sitting, feet supported, arms crossed to opposite shoulders.

Therapist: Standing at the patient's side.

Palpate: With the lateral aspect of the MCP joint of the index finger of the dorsal hand, palpate the spinous process of the caudal vertebra. For the upper thoracic region, the ventral hand is wound through the patient's crossed arms to rest on the contralateral shoulder. For the lower joints, the ventral hand is placed on the contralateral scapula, the arm resting against the patient's chest.

Localization: Flex the thorax until movement is perceived at the desired joint complex.

Mobilization: Fix the caudal vertebra with the dorsal hand and passively flex the joint complex about the appropriate coronal axis.

Extension

The technique is identical to the above except that extension is employed instead of flexion.

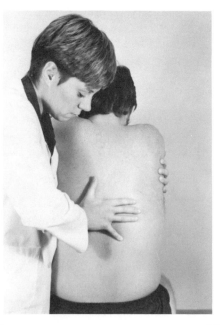

Notes:

A. SPINAL
1. PASSIVE ARTICULAR MOBILIZATION
b) Rotation/Sideflexion

Rotation is not a pure movement in the thoracic spine; it is conjoined with sideflexion. The most effective technique is therefore, the one which incorporates the appropriate sideflexion. The direction of 'ease of motion' must be located and the mobilization technique applied in this plane.

Patient: Sitting, feet supported, arms crossed to opposite shoulders.

Therapist: Standing at the patient's side.

Palpate: With the lateral aspect of the MCP joint of the index finger of the dorsal hand, palpate the spinous process of the caudal vertebra. For the upper thoracic region, the ventral hand is wound through the patient's crossed arms to rest on the contralateral shoulder. For the lower joints, the ventral hand is placed on the contralateral scapula, the arm resting against the patient's chest.

Mobilization: The direction of 'ease of motion' for rotation/side-flexion is located and the mobilization technique applied in this plane.

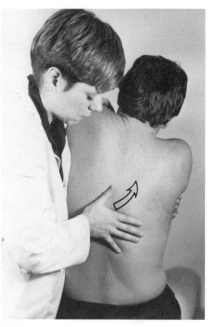

Notes:

A. SPINAL
1. PASSIVE ARTICULAR MOBILIZATION
c) Traction

Patient: Sitting, one hand on the contralateral shoulder, the other hand on the contralateral scapula.

Therapist: Standing behind the patient.

General Traction

Palpate: With both arms wrapped around the patient's trunk, grasp the patient's elbow which is closest to the chest. Grip the thorax with the inner arms.

Localization: Flex/extend the thorax to the desired level.

Mobilization: Apply traction by maintaining a firm grip on the thorax and straightening the knees.

Specific Traction

Palpate: Place a small towel which is rolled into a cylinder against the spinous process of the caudal vertebra of the joint complex. Fix the towel against the therapist's sternum. With both arms wrapped around the patient's trunk, grasp the patient's elbow which is closest to the chest. Grip the thorax with the inner arms.

Localization: Flex/extend the thorax to the desired level.

Mobilization: Apply traction by maintaining a firm grip on the thorax and gently straightening the knees.

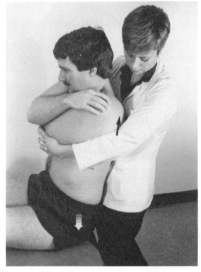

Notes:

_____

_____

_____

_____

_____

_____

_____

_____

_____

_____

_____

_____

_____

_____

_____

_____

_____

_____

_____

_____

_____

_____

A. SPINAL

1. PASSIVE ARTICULAR MOBILIZATION

d) Flexion/Rotation/Sideflexion

Patient:	Sidelying, head supported on a pillow, arms crossed to opposite shoulders.
Therapist:	Standing facing the patient.
Palpate:	With the tubercle of the scaphoid, palpate the transverse process of the caudal vertebra. With the palmar aspect of the head of the second metacarpal, palpate the contralateral transverse process of the cranial vertebra (dots). To control the thorax, grip the patient's crossed elbows with the other hand.
Localization:	Roll the patient supine over the mobilizing hand. Segmental localization is achieved by flexing and obliquely rotating/sideflexing the joint complex to the physiological limit with the hand controlling the thorax.
Mobilization:	Passively flex, rotate/sideflex the joint complex.

Extension/Rotation/Sideflexion

The technique is identical to the above except that extension is employed instead of flexion.

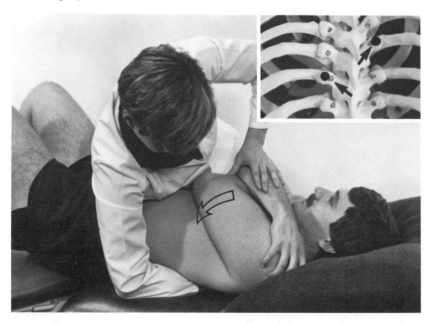

Notes:

_____

_____

_____

_____

_____

_____

_____

_____

_____

_____

_____

_____

_____

_____

_____

_____

_____

_____

_____

_____

_____

A. **SPINAL**
2. **ACTIVE MOBILIZATION**
   a) Flexion/Rotation/Sideflexion

Patient: Sitting, feet supported, arms crossed to opposite shoulders.

Therapist: Standing at the patient's side.

Palpate: With the index finger of the dorsal hand, palpate the interspinous space of the segment. Place the ventral hand on the contralateral shoulder.

Localization: The motion barrier is localized by flexing and obliquely rotating/sideflexing the joint complex to the physiological limit. Accurate localization is essential for the success of this technique.

Mobilization: From this position, the patient is instructed to hold the thorax still while the therapist applies a minimal force towards the midline. This isometric contraction is held for 3–5 seconds following which the patient is instructed to completely relax. The new flexion/rotation/sideflexion barrier is localized. The mobilization is repeated 3 times.

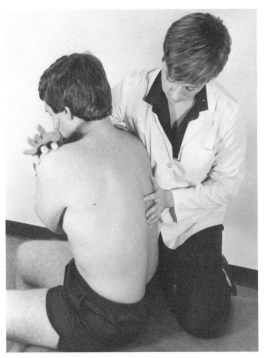

Notes:

A. **SPINAL**

2. **ACTIVE MOBILIZATION**

  b) Extension/Rotation/Sideflexion

Patient:	Sitting, feet supported, arms crossed to opposite shoulders.
Therapist:	Standing at the patient's side.
Palpate:	With the index finger of the dorsal hand, palpate the interspinous space of the segment. Place the ventral hand on the contralateral shoulder.
Localization:	The motion barrier is localized by extending and obliquely rotating/sideflexing the joint complex to the physiological limit. Accurate localization is essential for the success of this technique.
Mobilization:	From this position, the patient is instructed to hold the thorax still while the therapist applies a minimal force towards the midline. This isometric contraction is held for 3–5 seconds following which the patient is instructed to completely relax. The new extension/rotation/sideflexion barrier is localized. The mobilization is repeated 3 times.

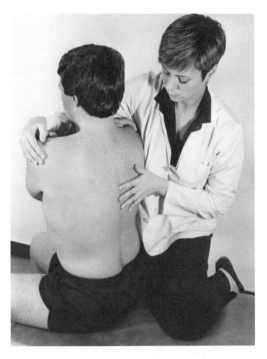

Notes:

_____

_____

_____

_____

_____

_____

_____

_____

_____

_____

_____

_____

_____

_____

_____

_____

_____

_____

_____

_____

_____

_____

_____

B. **COSTAL**

1. **PASSIVE ARTICULAR MOBILIZATION**

    a) Posteroanterior Pressures (P/A's)

Patient:	Prone.
Therapist:	Standing at the patient's side.
Palpate:	With the pisiform bone of the caudal hand, palpate the rib just lateral to the tubercle and medial to the angle. The fingers of this hand are directed cranially. With the pisiform bone of the cranial hand, palpate the contralateral transverse process of the thoracic vertebra to which the rib attaches. The fingers of this hand are directed caudally.
Localization:	To fix the spine, apply a posteroanterior pressure with the cranial hand to the transverse process of the thoracic vertebra.
Mobilization:	To distract the joint, apply an anterolateral pressure to the rib. To anteriorly glide the joint, apply a posteroanterior pressure along the line of the neck of the rib.

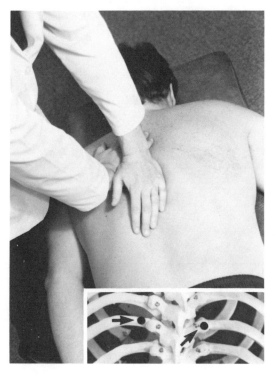

Notes:

_____

_____

_____

_____

_____

_____

_____

_____

_____

_____

_____

_____

_____

_____

_____

_____

_____

_____

_____

_____

_____

B. **COSTAL**

2. **ACTIVE MOBILIZATION**

   a) Inspiration

Patient:	Supine, the dorsum of the forearm on the side of the rib lesion resting against the patient's forehead.
Therapist:	Standing on the opposite side of the rib lesion facing the patient's head.
Palpate:	With the index, long and ring fingers, palpate the rib dorsally just lateral to the tubercle. Hook these fingers over the cranial border of the rib. The opposite hand rests on the medial aspect of the patient's elevated elbow.
Mobilization:	The patient is instructed to inspire fully while the therapist applies caudal pressure to the cranial aspect of the rib. At full inspiration, the patient is instructed to hold the elbow still against the therapist's gentle resistance (arrow). This isometric contraction is held for 3–5 seconds following which the patient is instructed to completely relax. The caudal pressure on the cranial aspect of the rib is maintained. The mobilization is repeated 3 times.

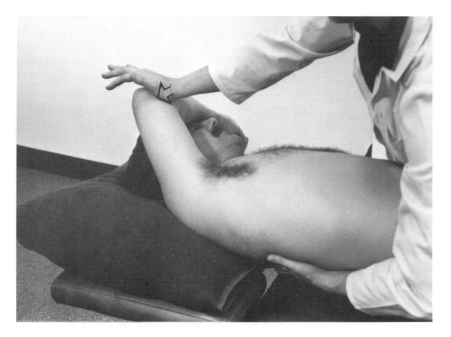

Notes:

B. **COSTAL**
2. **ACTIVE MOBILIZATION**
   b) Expiration

Patient:	Supine.
Therapist:	Standing at the patient's head facing the shoulders.
Palpate:	With the index finger, palpate the intercostal space caudal to the lesioned rib. For ribs 3–5: the other hand supports the cranium dorsally. For ribs 6–10: the other hand supports the thorax dorsally.
Localization:	Flex the neck/thorax (pump handle motion) or side-flex the neck/thorax (bucket handle motion) until the movement is perceived at the caudal intercostal space.
Mobilization:	The patient is instructed to breath out while the therapist increases flexion/sideflexion of the thorax. At full expiration, the patient is instructed to hold the head/thorax still against the therapist's resistance (arrow). This isometric contraction is held for 3–5 seconds following which the patient is instructed to completely relax. The new barrier is localized. The mobilization is repeated 3 times.

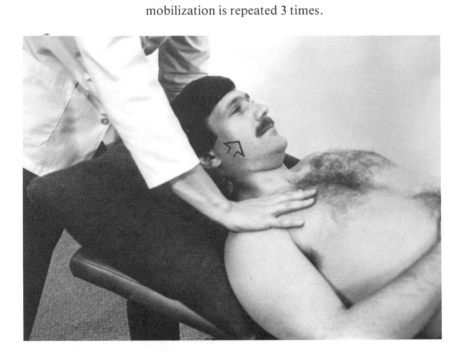

Notes:

Lumbar Region
T12–L1 to L5–S1

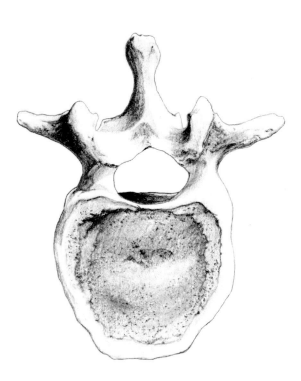

Lumbar Region — T12–L1 to L5–S1

Assessment

1. POSITIONAL TESTS

a) Hyperflexion

Patient:	Sitting, feet supported, lumbar spine fully flexed.
Therapist:	Standing behind the patient.
Palpate:	With the thumbs, palpate the spinous process of the T12 vertebra. From the tip of the spinous process, slide laterally and palpate the transverse processes.
Test:	Assess the position of the T12 vertebra relative to L1 by noting which transverse process is the most dorsal. A dorsal left transverse process of T12 relative to L1 is indicative of a left rotated position of the T12–L1 joint complex in hyperflexion.

Repeat this test for each segment.

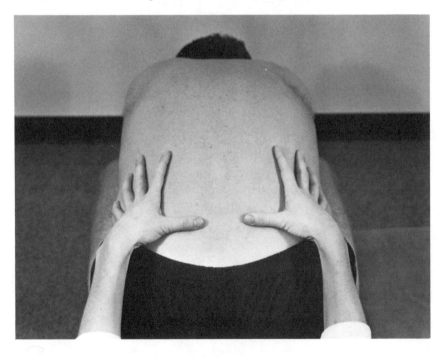

Notes:

1. POSITIONAL TESTS

b) Hyperextension

Patient: Prone, lumbar spine fully extended, chin resting in the hands.

Therapist: Standing at the patient's side.

Palpate: With the thumbs, palpate the spinous process of the T12 vertebra. From the tip of the spinous process slide laterally and palpate the transverse processes.

Test: Assess the position of the T12 vertebra relative to L1 by noting which transverse process is the most dorsal. A dorsal left transverse process of T12 relative to L1 is indicative of a left rotated position of the T12–L1 joint complex in hyperextension.

Repeat this test for each segment.

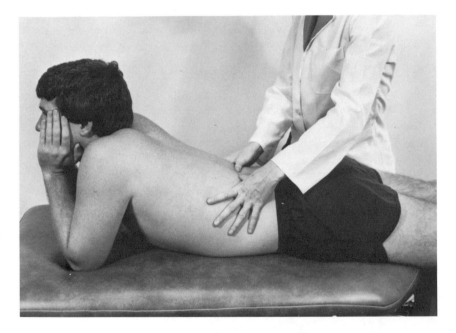

Notes:

_____

_____

_____

_____

_____

_____

_____

_____

_____

_____

_____

_____

_____

_____

_____

_____

_____

_____

_____

_____

_____

_____

_____

2. MOBILITY TESTS — Specific Articular Mobility

a) Active Physiological Mobility Tests

Patient:	Sitting, feet supported.
Therapist:	Standing behind the patient.
Palpate:	With the thumbs, palpate the transverse processes of the T12 vertebra.
Test:	a) Instruct the patient to flex the spine forward and note the cranial/ventral displacement of the transverse processes. Asymmetry *may* be indicative of dysfunction.
	b) Instruct the patient to extend the spine and note the caudal/dorsal displacement of the transverse processes. Asymmetry *may* be indicative of dysfunction.

Repeat these tests for each segment.

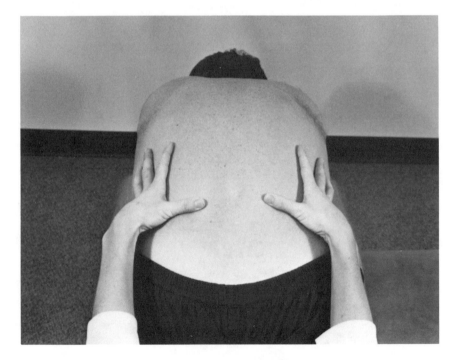

Notes:

2. MOBILITY TESTS — Specific Articular Mobility
b) Passive Physiological Mobility Tests
1. Flexion/Extension

Patient: Sidelying, close to the edge of the table, hips and knees flexed and supported on the therapist's abdomen.

Therapist: Standing facing the patient.

Palpate: With the caudal hand, support the patient's legs. With the index finger of the cranial hand, palpate the interspinous space of the segment.

Test: Passively flex/extend the joint complex about the appropriate coronal axis and note the quantity and quality of motion.

Repeat this test for each segment.

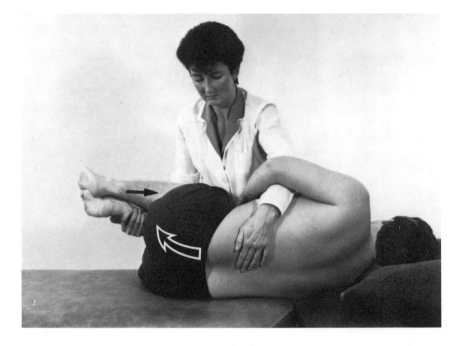

Notes:

2. MOBILITY TESTS — Specific Articular Mobility

b) Passive Physiological Mobility Tests

2. Sideflexion

a) Method A — Sidelying

Patient: Sidelying, close to the edge of the table, hips and knees flexed and supported on the therapist's abdomen.

Therapist: Standing facing the patient.

Palpate: With the index and middle fingers of the cranial hand, palpate the lateral aspect of the interspinous space. With the caudal hand, grasp the patient's lower legs proximal to the talocrural joints.

Test: Lean backwards to passively sideflex the joint complex about the appropriate sagittal axis. Note the quantity and quality of motion.

Repeat this test for each segment.

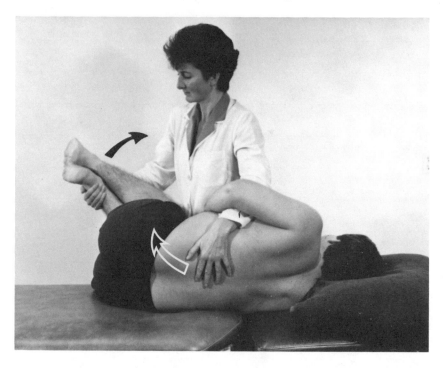

Notes:

_____

_____

_____

_____

_____

_____

_____

_____

_____

_____

_____

_____

_____

_____

_____

_____

_____

_____

_____

_____

_____

2. MOBILITY TESTS — Specific Articular Mobility
b) Passive Physiological Mobility Tests
2. Sideflexion
b) Method B — Prone

Patient: Prone with one knee flexed.

Therapist: Standing at the patient's side.

Palpate: With the caudal hand, support the anterior aspect of the distal thigh. With the index finger of the cranial hand, palpate the lateral aspect of the interspinous space of the segment.

Test: Passively abduct the patient's hip joint to the physiological limit. Further abduction sideflexes the lumbar spine. Note the quantity and quality of motion.

Repeat this test for each segment.

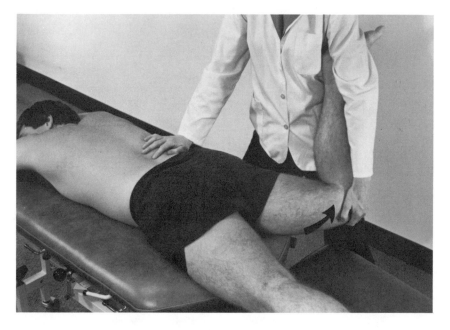

Notes:

2. **MOBILITY TESTS — Specific Articular Mobility**
   b) Passive Physiological Mobility Tests
      3. Sideflexion/Rotation
      Rotation is conjoined with sideflexion in this region of the spine and
      therefore a combined mobility test is required.

   Patient: Sidelying, close to the edge of the table, hips and knees
                      flexed.

   Therapist: Standing facing the patient.

   Palpate: With the index finger of the cranial hand, palpate the
                      interspinous space of the segment. The forearm rests
                      against the pectoral region. With the index finger of
                      the caudal hand, palpate the lateral aspect of the
                      interspinous space. The forearm rests against the pel-
                      vic girdle.

   Test: Passively sideflex/rotate the joint complex about the
                      appropriate oblique axis. Note the quantity and qual-
                      ity of motion.

                      Repeat this test for each segment.

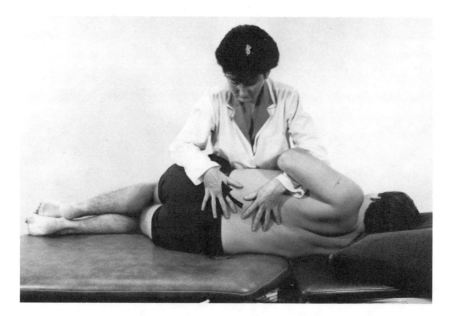

Notes:

_____

_____

_____

_____

_____

_____

_____

_____

_____

_____

_____

_____

_____

_____

_____

_____

_____

_____

_____

_____

_____

_____

2. MOBILITY TESTS — Specific Articular Mobility

   c) Passive Accessory Mobility Tests

      1. Posteroanterior Pressures (P/A's)

      a) Hyperflexion

Patient: Sitting, feet supported, lumbar spine fully flexed.

Therapist: Standing behind the patient.

Palpate: With the thumbs, palpate the transverse process of the T12 vertebra.

Test: Apply a posteroanterior pressure unilaterally to the transverse process of the T12 vertebra. Note the quantity and quality of motion.

               Repeat this test bilaterally for each segment.

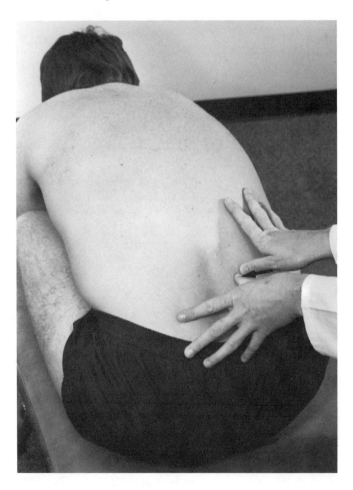

Notes:

2. MOBILITY TESTS — Specific Articular Mobility

c) Passive Accessory Mobility Tests

   1. Posteroanterior Pressures (P/A's)

   b) Hyperextension

Patient:	Prone, lumbar spine fully extended, chin resting in the hands.
Therapist:	Standing at the patient's side.
Palpate:	With the thumbs, palpate the transverse process of the T12 vertebra.
Test:	Apply a posteroanterior pressure unilaterally to the transverse process of the T12 vertebra. Note the quantity and quality of motion.

                  Repeat this test bilaterally for each segment.

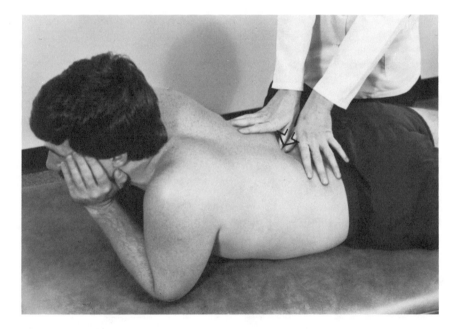

Notes:

3. **STRESS TESTS**
    a) Compression

Patient:	Supine, the hips and knees fully flexed.
Therapist:	Standing at the patient's side.
Palpate:	With the cranial arm, cradle the patient's knees to control the degree of hip and knee flexion. With the caudal hand, grip the patient's heels.
Test:	With the caudal hand, apply a compressive force cranially through the patient's heels. The direction of the force should be parallel to the floor. Note the quantity and quality of motion.

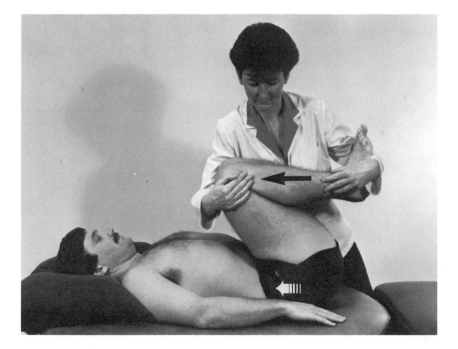

Notes:

3. STRESS TESTS

b) General Torsion

Patient:	Prone.
Therapist:	Standing facing the patient.
Palpate:	With the heel of the cranial hand palpate the thoracolumbar junction. With the caudal hand, grasp the contralateral innominate bone.
Test:	Fix the thoracolumbar junction and passively rotate the lumbar spine by lifting the contralateral innominate bone dorsally. Note the quantity and quality of motion.

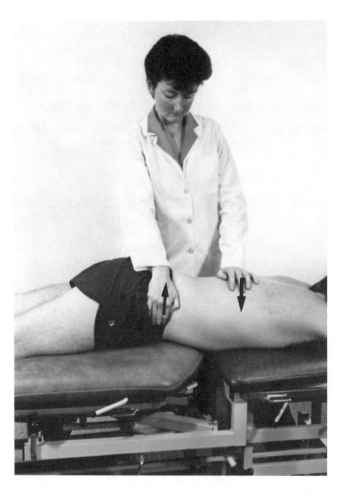

Notes:

3. STRESS TESTS

c) Specific Torsion

Patient: Sidelying, close to the edge of the table, hips and knees flexed.

Therapist: Standing facing the patient.

Palpate: With the thumb of the cranial hand, palpate the lateral aspect (top) of the spinous process of the cranial vertebra. The forearm rests against the pectoral region. With the index and long fingers of the caudal hand, palpate the lateral aspect (bottom) of the spinous process of the caudal vertebra. The forearm rests against the pelvic girdle.

Test: Passively rotate the segment (arrow) about a vertical axis. *This is an unphysiological movement.* Note the quantity and quality of motion.

Repeat this test bilaterally for each segment.

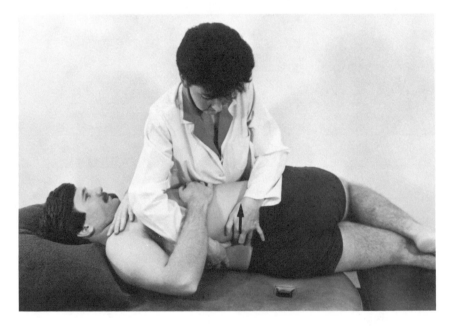

Notes:

_____

_____

_____

_____

_____

_____

_____

_____

_____

_____

_____

_____

_____

_____

_____

_____

_____

_____

_____

_____

_____

_____

3. STRESS TESTS

   d) Dorsal

Patient:	Sidelying, close to the edge of the table, hips and knees flexed and supported on the therapist's abdomen.
Therapist:	Standing facing the patient.
Palpate:	With the index finger of the cranial hand, palpate the interspinous space of the L5–S1 segment. With the caudal hand, support the patient's legs. Ensure that the segment is in a neutral position.
Test:	Dorsally shear the sacrum on the L5 vertebra by applying a dorsal force to the femora through the patient's flexed knees. Note the quantity and quality of motion.

Repeat this test for each segment.

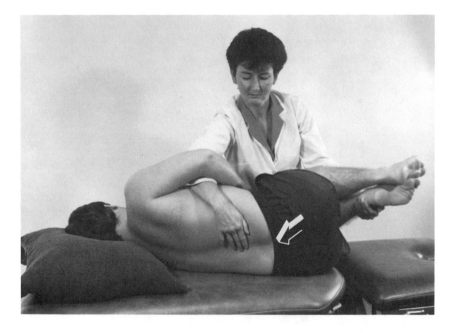

Notes:

3. STRESS TESTS

    e) Ventral

Patient:	Prone.
Therapist:	Standing at the patient's side.
Palpate:	With the pisiform bone of one hand, palpate the spinous process. Reinforce this hand with the other.
Test:	Apply a slow, steady, anterior shear to the segment through straight arms. Note the quantity and quality of motion.

Repeat this test for each segment.

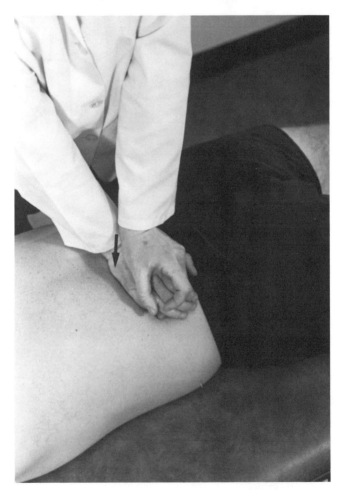

Notes:

_____

_____

_____

_____

_____

_____

_____

_____

_____

_____

_____

_____

_____

_____

_____

_____

_____

_____

_____

_____

_____

1. PASSIVE SOFT TISSUE MOBILIZATION

Patient: Sidelying on the side opposite that of the tissue to be mobilized.

Therapist: Standing facing the patient.

Palpate: With the forearms resting on the patient's lateral thorax and pelvic girdle and the fingers flexed in a lumbrical grip, palpate the soft tissue of the uppermost side.

Mobilization: The tight soft tissue is lifted up and stretched longitudinally as the therapist simultaneously adducts the shoulders and flexes the elbows. The hands are maintained in a loose lumbrical grip in order to avoid point pressure. Repeat the mobilization several times.

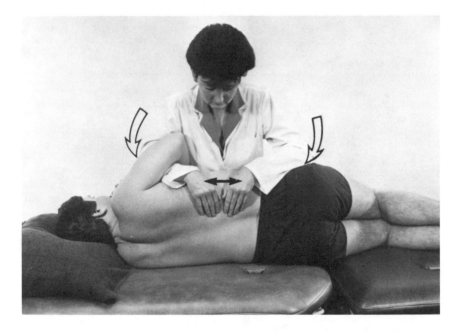

Notes:

_____

_____

_____

_____

_____

_____

_____

_____

_____

_____

_____

_____

_____

_____

_____

_____

_____

_____

_____

_____

2. PASSIVE ARTICULAR MOBILIZATION

a) General Traction

Patient:	Crook lying, close to the end of the table.
Therapist:	Standing at the end of the table facing the patient.
Palpate:	With the fingers interlaced, place the hands on the posterior aspect of the patient's proximal calves.
Mobilization:	A longitudinal traction force is applied to the lumbar spine by leaning backwards and pulling through the hands. The angle of pull may be altered in accordance with the level being treated and the patient's response.

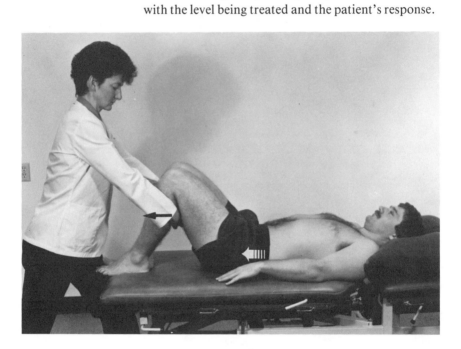

Notes:

_____

_____

_____

_____

_____

_____

_____

_____

_____

_____

_____

_____

_____

_____

_____

_____

_____

_____

_____

_____

_____

_____

2. PASSIVE ARTICULAR MOBILIZATION

b) Specific Traction

Patient:	Sidelying, close to the edge of the table.
Therapist:	Standing facing the patient.
Palpate and localization:	With the index finger of the caudal hand, palpate the interspinous space of the level *above* that to be treated. With the cranial hand, rotate the thoracolumbar spine caudally through the patient's lower arm to the level *above* that being treated. With the caudal hand, flex the patient's top hip joint until full flexion has been reached at the level *below* that being treated. The interspinous space of this segment is palpated by the index finger of the cranial hand, the forearm of which is supporting the thorax. Allow the foot of this leg to rest in the popliteal fossa of the lower leg whilst maintaining support of the knee. Instruct the patient to stretch the lower leg towards the end of the table. Support the pelvic girdle with the caudal forearm. The therapist's *lower* lateral costal region should be in contact with the patient's pelvic girdle.
Mobilization:	The fingers of both hands should be free to palpate the interspinous space of the segment to be tractioned or to adjust the segmental localization if necessary. Traction is applied to the segment via a straight caudal force against the patient's pelvic girdle with the therapist's lower lateral thorax. The cranial arm stabilizes the patient's thorax.

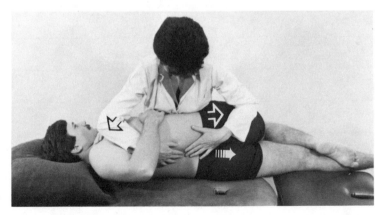

Notes:

2. PASSIVE ARTICULAR MOBILIZATION

c) Sideflexion/Rotation

Rotation is conjoined with sideflexion in this region of the spine and a combined technique is the most effective. Pure rotation as a treatment technique is detrimental to the health of the joint since this motion is unphysiological.

Patient:	Sidelying, close to the edge of the table.
Therapist:	Standing facing the patient.
Palpate and localization:	With the index finger of the caudal hand, palpate the interspinous space of the level *above* that to be treated. With the cranial hand, rotate the thoraco-lumbar spine caudally through the patient's lower arm to the level *above* that being treated. With the caudal hand, flex the patient's top hip joint until full flexion has been reached at the level *below* that being treated. The interspinous space of this segment is palpated by the index finger of the cranial hand, the forearm of which is supporting the thorax. Allow the foot of this leg to rest in the popliteal fossa of the lower leg. Instruct the patient to stretch the lower leg towards the end of the table. Support the pelvic girdle with the caudal forearm.
Mobilization:	The fingers of both hands should be free to palpate the interspinous space of the segment being treated. The direction of 'ease of motion' for sideflexion/rotation is located and the mobilization technique applied in this plane.

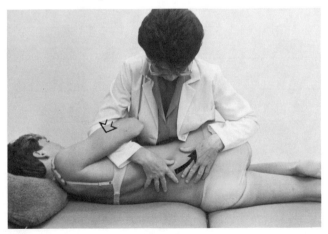

Notes:

_____

_____

_____

_____

_____

_____

_____

_____

_____

_____

_____

_____

_____

_____

_____

_____

_____

_____

_____

_____

_____

3. ACTIVE MOBILIZATION

a) Extension/Rotation/Sideflexion

1. Method A — Sidelying

Patient: Sidelying, close to the edge of the table.

Therapist: Standing facing the patient.

Palpate and localization: With the index finger of the caudal hand, palpate the interspinous space of the level *above* that to be treated. With the cranial hand, rotate the thoraco-lumbar spine caudally through the patient's lower arm to the level *above* that being treated. Fix this rotation component with the forearm of the cranial hand. Palpate the interspinous space of the level *below* that being treated with the index finger of the cranial hand. With the caudal hand, flex the patient's top hip joint until full flexion has been reached at the level *below* that being treated.

Segmental Localization: The segmental motion barrier is localized by extending and obliquely rotating/sideflexing the joint complex to the physiological limit. Accurate localization is essential for the success of this technique.

Mobilization: From this position, the patient is instructed to hold still while the therapist applies a gentle resistance to the pelvic girdle (arrow). This isometric contraction recruits the segmental spinal stabilizers which can be monitored by the fingers of the cranial hand. The contraction is held for 3–5 seconds following which the patient is instructed to completely relax. The new barrier of extension/rotation/sideflexion is localized. The mobilization is repeated 3 times.

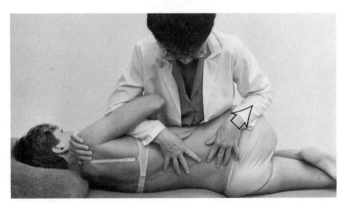

Notes:

_____

_____

_____

_____

_____

_____

_____

_____

_____

_____

_____

_____

_____

_____

_____

_____

_____

_____

_____

_____

_____

_____

3. ACTIVE MOBILIZATION
a) Extension/Rotation/Sideflexion
2. Method B — Sitting

Patient: Sitting, feet supported, arms crossed to opposite shoulders.

Therapist: Standing at the patient's side.

Palpate: With the index finger of the dorsal hand, palpate the interspinous space of the segment. Place the ventral hand on the contralateral shoulder.

Localization: The motion barrier is localized by extending and obliquely rotating/sideflexing the joint complex to the physiological limit. Accurate localization is essential for the success of this technique.

Mobilization: From this position, the patient is instructed to hold still while the therapist applies a minimal force to the shoulder girdle (arrow). This isometric contraction is held for 3–5 seconds following which the patient is instructed to completely relax. The new extension/rotation/sideflexion barrier is localized. The mobilization is repeated 3 times.

This technique can also be used for flexion/rotation/sideflexion employing flexion instead of extension.

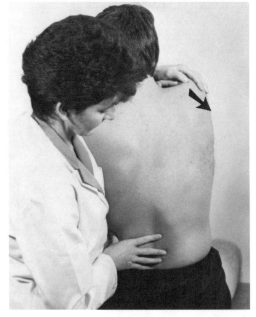

Notes:

3. ACTIVE MOBILIZATION

b) Flexion/Rotation/Sideflexion

1. Method A

Patient: Sidelying, close to the edge of the table.

Therapist: Standing facing the patient.

Palpate and localization: With the index finger of the caudal hand, palpate the interspinous space of the level *above* that to be treated. With the cranial hand, rotate the thoracolumbar spine caudally through the patient's lower arm to the level *above* that being treated. Fix this rotation component with the forearm of the cranial hand. Palpate the interspinous space of the level *below* that being treated with the index finger of the cranial hand. With the caudal hand, flex the patient's top hip joint until full flexion has been reached at the level *below* that being treated.

Segmental Localization: The segmental motion barrier is localized by flexing and obliquely rotating/sideflexing the joint complex to the physiological limit. Accurate localization is essential for the success of this technique.

Mobilization: From this position, the patient is instructed to hold still while the therapist applies a gentle resistance to the pelvic girdle (arrow). This isometric contraction recruits the segmental spinal stabilizers which can be monitored by the fingers of the cranial hand. The contraction is held for 3–5 seconds following which the patient is instructed to completely relax. The new barrier of flexion/rotation/sideflexion is localized. The mobilization is repeated 3 times.

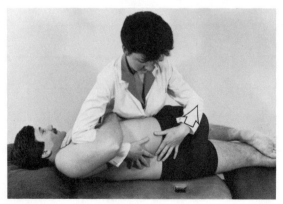

Notes:

_____

_____

_____

_____

_____

_____

_____

_____

_____

_____

_____

_____

_____

_____

_____

_____

_____

_____

_____

_____

_____

3. ACTIVE MOBILIZATION

b) Flexion/Rotation/Sideflexion

2. Method B

Patient:	Sidelying, close to the edge of the table.
Therapist:	Standing facing the patient.
Palpate and localization:	With the index finger of the caudal hand, palpate the interspinous space of the level *above* that to be treated. With the cranial hand, rotate the thoraco-lumbar spine caudally through the patient's lower arm to the level *above* that being treated. Fix this rotation component with the forearm of the cranial hand. Palpate the interspinous space of the level *below* that being treated with the index finger of the cranial hand. With the caudal hand, flex the patient's top hip joint until full flexion has been reached at the level *below* that being treated. The patient's top leg is supported on the therapist's abdomen.
Segmental localization:	The segmental motion barrier is localized by flexing and obliquely rotating/sideflexing the joint complex to the physiological limit using the patient's flexed top leg as the lever.
Mobilization:	From this position, the patient is instructed to hold still while the therapist applies a gentle resistance to the leg (arrow). This isometric contraction recruits the segmental spinal stabilizers which can be monitored by the fingers of the cranial hand. The contraction is held for 3–5 seconds following which the patient is instructed to completely relax. The new barrier of flexion/rotation/sideflexion is localized using the leg. The mobilization is repeated 3 times.

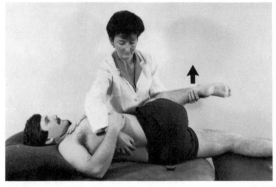

Notes:

_____

_____

_____

_____

_____

_____

_____

_____

_____

_____

_____

_____

_____

_____

_____

_____

_____

_____

_____

_____

_____

3. ACTIVE MOBILIZATION

c) Multisegmental Myofascial Stretch

Patient: Sitting, feet supported, arms crossed to opposite shoulders.

Therapist: Standing beside the patient on the side of the concavity of the multisegmental curve.

Palpate: With the index finger of the dorsal hand, palpate the segmental musculature at the apex of the curve. The ventral hand is placed on the contralateral scapula, the arm resting against the patient's chest.

Localization: With the spine in a neutral position, localize the side flexion and rotation barriers by sideflexing the spine towards the convexity of the curve until motion is perceived at the apex, then rotating the spine away from the convexity until the motion is again perceived at the apex. The multisegmental myofascia on the side of the concavity is now on stretch.

Mobilization: From this position, the patient is instructed to hold still while the therapist applies a resistance to the shoulder girdle (arrow). The contraction may be isometric, isotonic or isolytic and is held for 3–5 seconds following which the patient is instructed to completely relax. The new barrier is localized. The mobilization is repeated 3 times.

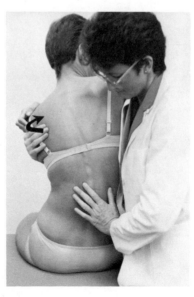

Notes:

_____

_____

_____

_____

_____

_____

_____

_____

_____

_____

_____

_____

_____

_____

_____

_____

_____

_____

_____

_____

_____

Pelvic Girdle Region

Sacroiliac Joints and Pubic Symphysis

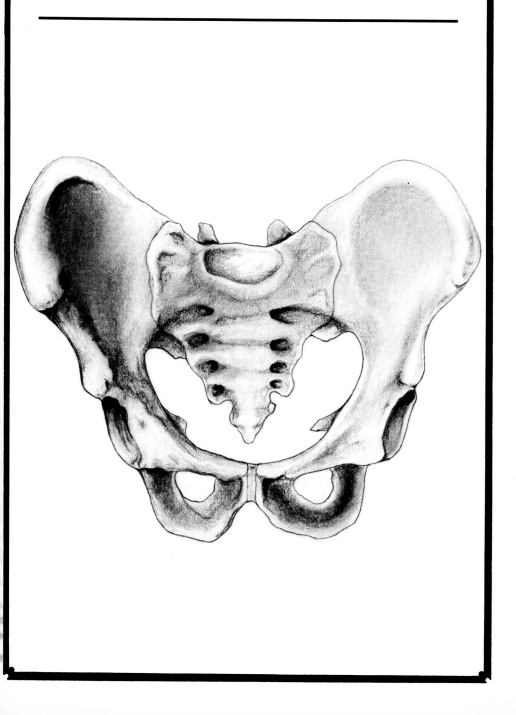

Pelvic Girdle Region — Sacroiliac Joints and Pubic Symphysis

1. POSITIONAL TESTS

    a) Innominate

        1.   Iliac Crest

Patient: Supine.

Therapist: Standing at the patient's side.

Palpate: With the radial border of the index fingers, palpate the lateral aspect of the iliac crest bilaterally. Move the soft tissue overlying the iliac crest medially and cranially so that the index fingers rest on the highest point of the iliac crest. Using peripheral vision, compare the craniocaudal relationship of the 2 sides.

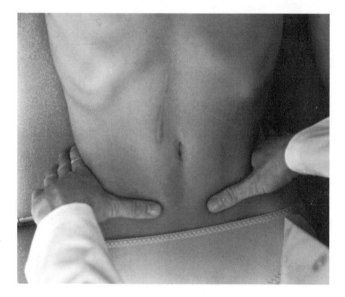

Notes:

_____

_____

_____

_____

_____

_____

_____

_____

_____

_____

_____

_____

_____

_____

_____

_____

_____

_____

_____

_____

_____

1. **POSITIONAL TESTS**
   a) Innominate
      2. Anterior Superior Iliac Spine (ASIS)
      a) craniocaudal

Patient:	Supine.
Therapist:	Standing at the patient's side.
Palpate:	Initially, palpate the ASIS through the soft tissue with the heel of the hand. Then using the thumbs, palpate the caudal aspect of the ASIS bilaterally. Using peripheral vision, compare the craniocaudal relationship of the 2 sides.

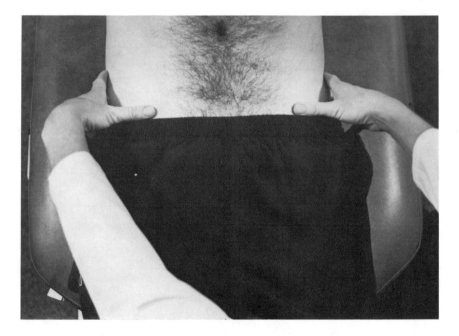

Notes:

_____

_____

_____

_____

_____

_____

_____

_____

_____

_____

_____

_____

_____

_____

_____

_____

_____

_____

_____

_____

_____

1. **POSITIONAL TESTS**
   a) Innominate
      2. Anterior Superior Iliac Spine (ASIS)
      b) mediolateral

   Patient: Supine.

   Therapist: Standing at the patient's side.

   Palpate: Initially, palpate the ASIS through the soft tissue with the heel of the hand. Then using the thumbs, palpate the medial aspect of the ASIS bilaterally. Using peripheral vision, compare the mediolateral relationship of the ASIS to the midline of the body, ie: the xyphoid process, umbilicus or pubic symphysis.

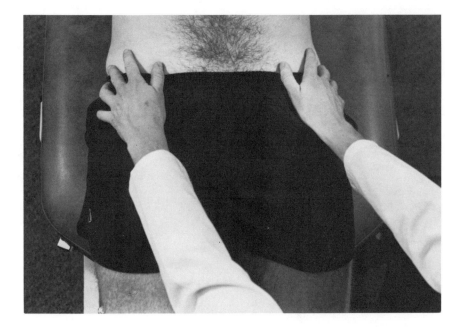

Notes:

_____

_____

_____

_____

_____

_____

_____

_____

_____

_____

_____

_____

_____

_____

_____

_____

_____

_____

_____

1. POSITIONAL TESTS

a) Innominate Bone

3. Pubic Tubercle

Patient: Supine.

Therapist: Standing at the patient's side.

Palpate: Initially, palpate the pubic symphysis through the soft tissue with the heel of the hand. Then using the thumbs, palpate the cranial aspect of the pubic tubercles which are approximately 1cm. apart and cranial to the pubic symphysis. Compare the craniocaudal relationship of the 2 sides.

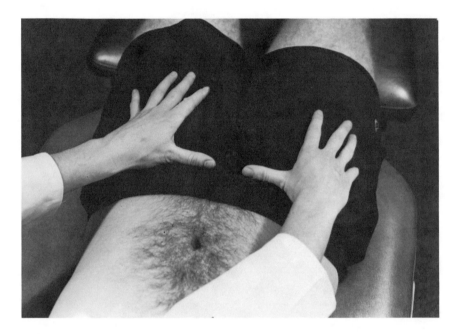

Notes:

_____

_____

_____

_____

_____

_____

_____

_____

_____

_____

_____

_____

_____

_____

_____

_____

_____

_____

_____

_____

_____

1. POSITIONAL TESTS

a) Innominate

4. Posterior Superior Iliac Spine (PSIS)

Patient: Prone.

Therapist: Standing at the patient's side. Observe the "dimple". The PSIS lies approximately 1 cm. caudal to the dimple.

Palpate: With the thumbs, palpate the caudal aspect of the PSIS bilaterally. Using peripheral vision, compare the craniocaudal relationship of the 2 sides.

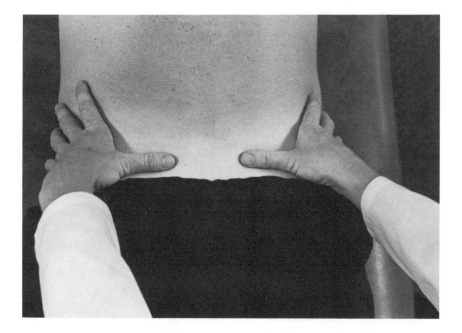

Notes:

_____

_____

_____

_____

_____

_____

_____

_____

_____

_____

_____

_____

_____

_____

_____

_____

_____

_____

_____

_____

_____

_____

_____

_____

_____

1. POSITIONAL TESTS

a) Innominate

5. Ischial Tuberosity

Patient: Prone.

Therapist: Standing at the patient's side.

Palpate: Initially, palpate the ischial tuberosity through the soft tissue at the gluteal fold with the heel of the hand. Then using the thumbs, palpate the most caudal aspect of the tuberosity bilaterally. Compare the craniocaudal relationship of the 2 sides.

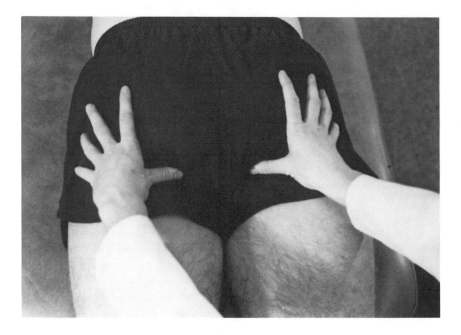

Notes:

_____

_____

_____

_____

_____

_____

_____

_____

_____

_____

_____

_____

_____

_____

_____

_____

_____

_____

_____

_____

_____

_____

1. POSITIONAL TESTS
b) Sacrum
1. Sacral Sulcus Depth

The sulcus depth is the vertical (dorsoventral) distance between the posterior superior iliac spine (PSIS) and the base of the sacrum.

Patient: Prone.

Therapist: Standing at the patient's side.

Palpate: With the thumbs, palpate the caudal aspect of the PSIS bilaterally. From this position, roll the thumbs medially and ventrally into the sacral sulcus. Palpate through the soft tissue to the base of the sacrum. Compare the relative depth of the 2 sides using palpatory sense rather than vision.

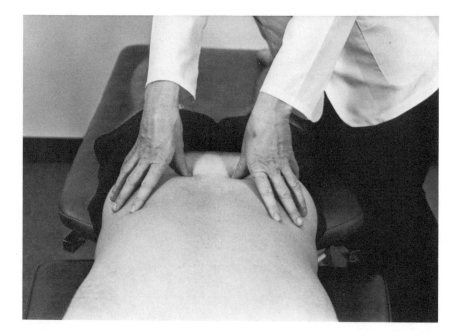

Notes:

_____

_____

_____

_____

_____

_____

_____

_____

_____

_____

_____

_____

_____

_____

_____

_____

_____

_____

_____

_____

_____

_____

1. POSITIONAL TESTS

b) Sacrum

2. Inferior Lateral Angle (ILA)

Patient: Prone.

Therapist: Standing at the patient's side.

Palpate: With the index finger, palpate the median sacral crest. Slide caudally along the spinous processes of the sacrum to the sacral hiatus. From this position, palpate laterally and caudally at an angle of 45° to the midline to reach the dorsal aspect of the inferior lateral angle. Compare the ventrodorsal relationship of the 2 sides.

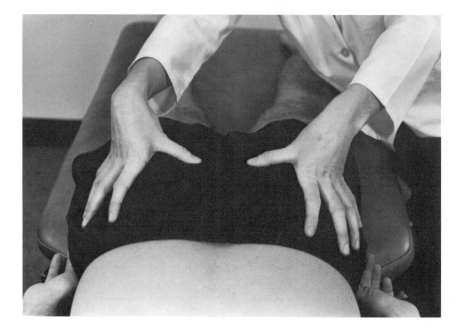

Notes:

_____

_____

_____

_____

_____

_____

_____

_____

_____

_____

_____

_____

_____

_____

_____

_____

_____

_____

_____

_____

2. SOFT TISSUE TENSION TEST

    a) Sacrotuberous Ligament

        Patient: Prone.

        Therapist: Standing at the patient's side.

        Palpate: With the heels of the hands, locate the ischial tuberosities through the soft tissue at the gluteal folds. Then with the thumbs, palpate the caudal aspect of the ischial tuberosities. From this point, slide medially and cranially to palpate the sacrotuberous ligament. Compare the relative tension of the left to the right side.

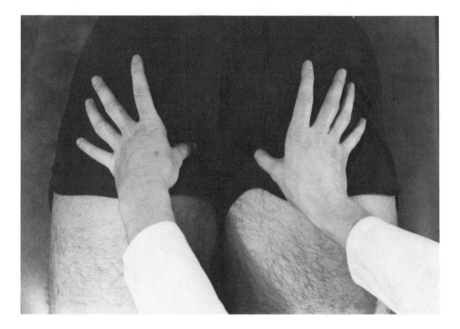

Notes:

_____

_____

_____

_____

_____

_____

_____

_____

_____

_____

_____

_____

_____

_____

_____

_____

_____

_____

_____

_____

_____

_____

_____

3. MOBILITY TESTS

a) Forward Bending Test — Standing

Patient:	Standing, feet directly under the hips, even distribution of body weight through both lower limbs.
Therapist:	Standing behind the patient.
Palpate:	With the thumbs, palpate the inferior aspect of the posterior superior iliac spine (PSIS) bilaterally.
Test:	Instruct the patient to bend forward keeping the knees extended. Observe and palpate the quality (symmetry) of the osteokinematic motion of both PSIS's, which should move equally in a cranial direction. This test is not specifically a sacroiliac articular mobility test, but rather a global test of lower quadrant function in forward bending. The mobility of the functional pelvic girdle in this test is influenced by: 1. the stability of the lumbar spine and the pelvic girdle under body weight. 2. the mobility of the lumbar, sacroiliac and hip joints. 3. the myofascial tension in the posterior aspect of the trunk, pelvis and lower limbs. 4. the functional length of the lower extremities. Asymmetry is indicative of dysfunction in the lower quadrant.

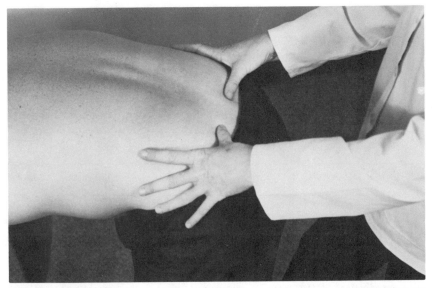

PELVIC GIRDLE REGION   ASSESSMENT

Notes:

3. MOBILITY TESTS

b) Forward Bending Test — Sitting

Patient: Sitting, feet supported.

Therapist: Standing behind the patient.

Palpate: With the thumbs, palpate the caudal aspect of the posterior superior iliac spine (PSIS) bilaterally.

Test: Instruct the patient to bend forward. Observe and palpate the quality (symmetry) of the osteokinematic motion of both PSIS's, which should move equally in a cranial direction. This test is not specifically a sacro-iliac articular mobility test, but rather a global test of lumbar/pelvic/hip function in forward bending. The mobility of the functional pelvic girdle in this test is predominately influenced by:

1. the mobility of the lumbar, sacroiliac and hip joints.

2. the myofascial tension in the posterior aspect of the trunk and pelvis.

Asymmetry is indicative of lumbar, pelvic girdle or hip dysfunction.

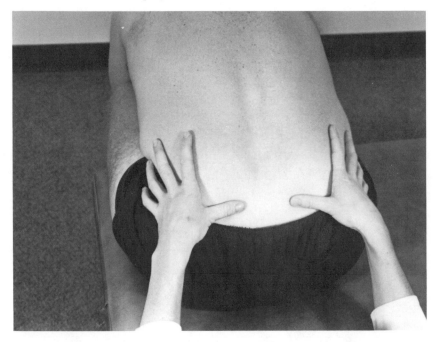

Notes:

3. **MOBILITY TESTS**

    c) Posteroanterior Pressures (P/A's)

        1. Inferior Lateral Angle

Patient: Prone.

Therapist: Standing at the patient's side.

Palpate: With the thumbs, palpate the sacral hiatus. From this position, slide the thumbs laterally and caudally at an angle of 45° to the midline to reach the dorsal aspect of the inferior lateral angle.

Test: Apply a posteroanterior pressure unilaterally and then bilaterally to the inferior lateral angle. The direction of the applied pressure is varied until the plane of the sacroiliac joint is found. Note the quantity and quality of motion.

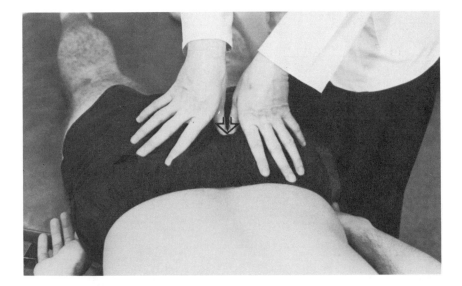

Notes:

_____

_____

_____

_____

_____

_____

_____

_____

_____

_____

_____

_____

_____

_____

_____

_____

_____

_____

_____

_____

3. **MOBILITY TESTS**

   c) Posteroanterior Pressures (P/A's)

     2. Sacral Base

     Patient: Prone.

     Therapist: Standing at the patient's side.

     Palpate: With the thumbs, palpate the sacral base directly lateral to the spinous process of S1.

     Test: Apply a posteroanterior pressure to the sacral base unilaterally and then bilaterally. The direction of the applied pressure is varied until the plane of the sacroiliac joint is found. Note the quantity and quality of motion.

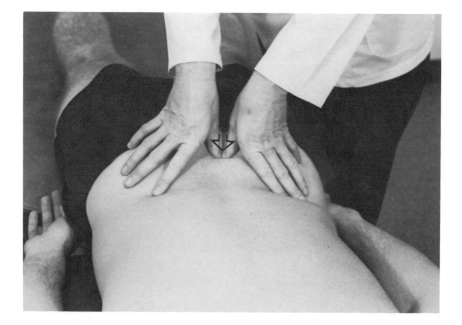

Notes:

_____

_____

_____

_____

_____

_____

_____

_____

_____

_____

_____

_____

_____

_____

_____

_____

_____

_____

_____

_____

_____

_____

3. MOBILITY TESTS

    d) Kinetic Test

       1. Ipsilateral

Patient:	Standing, feet directly under the hips, even distribution of body weight through both lower limbs.
Therapist:	Standing behind the patient.
Palpate:	With one thumb, palpate the caudal aspect of the posterior superior iliac spine (PSIS) of the joint being assessed. With the other thumb, palpate the median sacral crest at a point level with the PSIS.
Test:	Instruct the patient to flex the ipsilateral hip and knee to 90° and note the caudal displacement of the PSIS relative to the median sacral crest.
Addendum:	The pelvis should remain in its initial coronal and horizontal plane. Also note the patient's ability to balance on the weight bearing limb. In this posture, the line of gravity passes through the weight bearing sacroiliac joint to the arcuate line of the innominate bone and then to the hip joint. Sacroiliac joint dysfunction can potentially disrupt this weight transference and consequently alter the balance on that side.

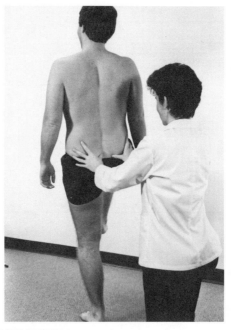

Notes:

_____

_____

_____

_____

_____

_____

_____

_____

_____

_____

_____

_____

_____

_____

_____

_____

_____

_____

_____

_____

_____

_____

_____

3. MOBILITY TESTS

d) Kinetic Test

2. Contralateral

Patient: Standing, feet directly under the hips, even distribution of body weight through both lower limbs.

Therapist: Standing behind the patient.

Palpate: With one thumb, palpate the caudal aspect of the posterior superior iliac spine (PSIS) of the joint being assessed. With the other thumb, palpate the median sacral crest at a point level with the PSIS.

Test: Instruct the patient to flex the contralateral hip and knee to 90° and note the caudal displacement of the median sacral crest relative to the PSIS.

Addendum: The pelvis should remain in its initial coronal and horizontal plane. Also note the patient's ability to balance on the weight bearing limb. In this posture, the line of gravity passes through the weight bearing sacroiliac joint to the arcuate line of the innominate bone and then to the hip joint. Sacroiliac joint dysfunction can potentially disrupt this weight transference and consequently alter the balance on that side.

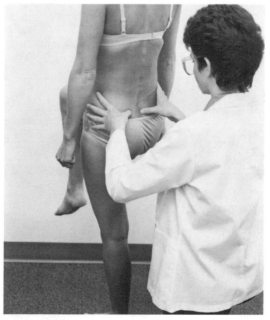

Notes:

_____

_____

_____

_____

_____

_____

_____

_____

_____

_____

_____

_____

_____

_____

_____

_____

_____

_____

_____

4. STRESS TESTS

a) Transverse Ventral

Patient: Supine.

Therapist: Standing at the patient's side.

Palpate: With crossed arms, palpate the medial aspect of the ASIS bilaterally with the heels of the hands.

Test: Apply a slow, steady force dorsolaterally through the ASIS's thus stressing the ventral sacroiliac ligament and indirectly, the transverse pubic ligament. Maintain this force for 20 seconds and note any symptoms.

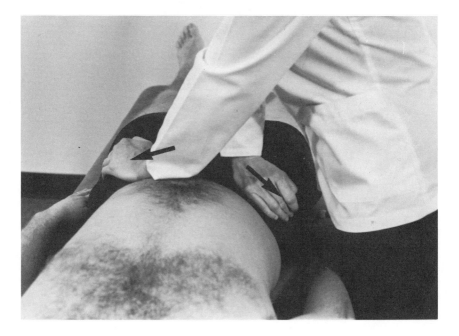

Notes:

_____

_____

_____

_____

_____

_____

_____

_____

_____

_____

_____

_____

_____

_____

_____

_____

_____

_____

_____

4. STRESS TESTS

b) Craniocaudal Pubic Symphysis

Patient:	Supine.
Therapist:	Standing at the patient's side.
Palpate:	With the heel of one hand, palpate the superior ramus of the pubis closest to the therapist. With the heel of the other hand, palpate the inferior ramus of the opposite pubis.
Test:	With both hands, apply a slow, steady, craniocaudal shear to the pubic symphysis noting any local symptoms. Switch hands and repeat the test.

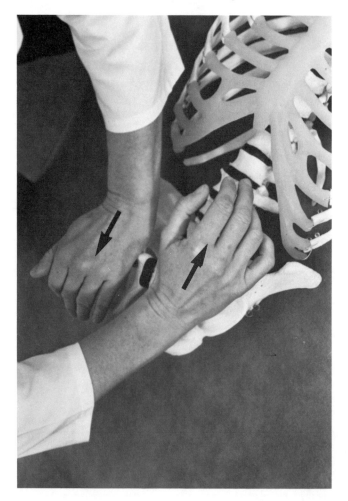

Notes:

_____

_____

_____

_____

_____

_____

_____

_____

_____

_____

_____

_____

_____

_____

_____

_____

_____

_____

_____

_____

4. STRESS TESTS

    c) Transverse Dorsal

Patient:	Sidelying, both hips and knees flexed.
Therapist:	Standing behind the patient.
Palpate:	With the heel of the hand, palpate the ventrolateral aspect of the iliac crest. Reinforce this hand with the other hand.
Test:	Apply a slow, steady pressure towards the table through the ventral aspect of the ilium. This stresses the dorsal aspect of the sacroiliac joint and the dorsal sacroiliac ligaments. Maintain this force for 20 seconds and note any symptoms.

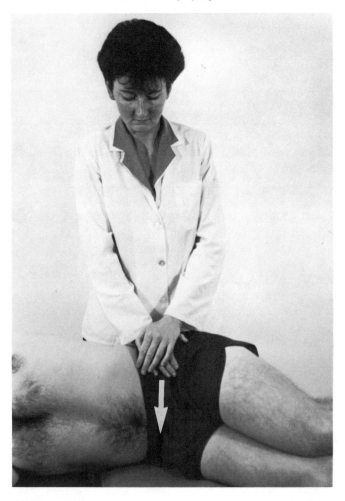

PELVIC GIRDLE REGION   ASSESSMENT

Notes:

_____

_____

_____

_____

_____

_____

_____

_____

_____

_____

_____

_____

_____

_____

_____

_____

_____

_____

_____

4. STRESS TESTS

d) Sacrotuberous Ligament

Patient:	Supine with the hip and knee flexed.
Therapist:	Standing at the patient's side.
Palpate:	Place the hands on top of the flexed knee with the fingers interlaced.
Test:	Flex and adduct the hip joint to the physiological limit. From this position, apply a longitudinal force along the line of the femur in an obliquely lateral direction. Maintain this force for 20 seconds and note any symptoms.

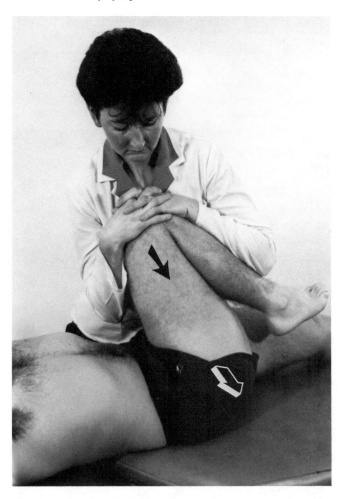

Notes:

_____

_____

_____

_____

_____

_____

_____

_____

_____

_____

_____

_____

_____

_____

_____

_____

_____

_____

_____

_____

_____

1. INNOMINATE

a) Superior Subluxation in Anterior Rotation

Patient: Prone.

Therapist: Standing at the end of the table facing the patient.

Palpate: With both hands, grasp the patient's lower leg, proximal to the talocrural joint, on the side being treated.

Localization: A caudal pull is applied to the lower extremity in varying degrees of hip abduction and extension to locate the position in which the greatest craniocaudal excursion of the sacroiliac joint occurs.

Mobilization: From this position, the motion barrier is reached by applying a longitudinal pull through the leg. An initial 'test pull' must be painless, if not, do not manipulate. If painless, a high velocity, low amplitude tug is applied through the leg to the sacroiliac joint.

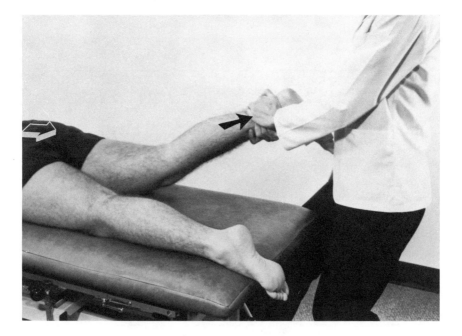

Notes:

_____

_____

_____

_____

_____

_____

_____

_____

_____

_____

_____

_____

_____

_____

_____

_____

_____

_____

_____

_____

1. INNOMINATE

   b) Superior Subluxation in Posterior Rotation

   Patient: Supine.

   Therapist: Standing at the end of the table facing the patient.

   Palpate: With both hands, grasp the patient's lower leg, proximal to the talocrural joint, on the side being treated.

   Localization: A caudal pull is applied to the lower extremity in varying degrees of hip abduction and flexion to locate the position in which the greatest craniocaudal excursion of the sacroiliac joint occurs.

   Mobilization: From this position, the motion barrier is reached by applying a longitudinal pull through the leg. An initial 'test pull' must be painless, if not, do not manipulate. If painless, a high velocity, low amplitude tug is applied through the leg to the sacroiliac joint.

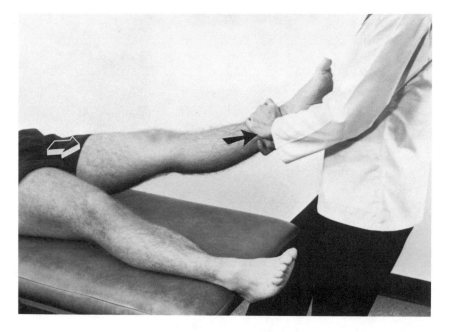

Notes:

_____

_____

_____

_____

_____

_____

_____

_____

_____

_____

_____

_____

_____

_____

_____

_____

_____

_____

_____

_____

_____

_____

1. INNOMINATE

c) Posterior Rotation

1. Method A – Prone

Patient: Prone.

Therapist: Standing at the patient's side.

Palpate: With the caudal hand, support the ventral aspect of the thigh just above the knee on the side of the lesion. With the heel of the cranial hand, palpate the PSIS of the innominate bone.

Localization: The motion barrier is localized by first extending the hip joint to the physiological limit. Further hip extension osteokinematically rotates the innominate anteriorly on the sacrum and this is continued until motion at the lumbosacral junction is perceived. The sacroiliac joint motion barrier has then been reached.

Mobilization: From this position, the patient is instructed to flex the hip against the therapist's resistance (arrow). This isometric contraction is held for 3–5 seconds following which the patient is instructed to completely relax. The new anterior rotation barrier is localized by further extension of the hip joint. The mobilization is repeated 3 times.

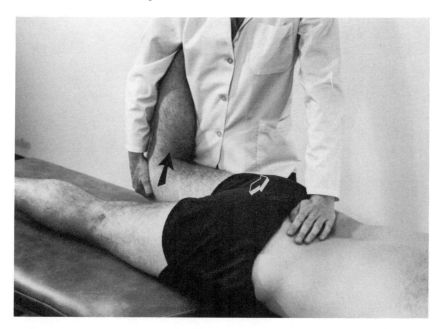

Notes:

_____

_____

_____

_____

_____

_____

_____

_____

_____

_____

_____

_____

_____

_____

_____

_____

_____

_____

1. INNOMINATE

   c) Posterior Rotation

     2. Method B — Sidelying

Patient: Sidelying, lower hip and knee fully flexed and held by the patient.

Therapist: Standing behind the patient.

Palpate: With the thumb of the cranial hand, palpate the sacral sulcus, allowing the rest of this hand to lie over the iliac crest. With the caudal hand, support the medial aspect of the uppermost flexed knee. The patient's lower leg rests on the therapist's forearm.

Localization: The motion barrier is localized by first extending the hip joint to the physiological limit. Further hip extension osteokinematically rotates the innominate anteriorly on the sacrum and this is continued until motion at the lumbosacral junction is perceived. The sacroiliac joint motion barrier has then been reached.

Mobilization: From this position, the patient is instructed to flex the hip against the therapist's resistance (arrow). This isometric contraction is held for 3–5 seconds following which the patient is instructed to completely relax. The new anterior rotation barrier is localized by further extension of the hip joint. The mobilization is repeated 3 times.

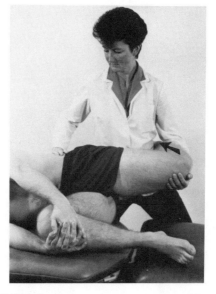

Notes:

_____

_____

_____

_____

_____

_____

_____

_____

_____

_____

_____

_____

_____

_____

_____

_____

_____

_____

_____

1. INNOMINATE

d) Anterior Rotation

Patient: Supine, hip and knee on the side of the lesion flexed.

Therapist: Standing at the patient's side.

Palpate: With one hand, cup the ischial tuberosity on the side of the lesion. With the index and long fingers of the other hand, palpate the lumbosacral junction and the sacral sulcus.

Localization: The motion barrier is localized by first flexing the hip joint to the physiological limit. Further hip flexion osteokinematically rotates the innominate posteriorly on the sacrum and this is continued until motion at the lumbosacral junction is perceived. The sacroiliac joint motion barrier has then been reached.

Mobilization: From this position, the patient is instructed to extend the hip against the resistance provided by the therapist's shoulder (arrow). This isometric contraction is held for 3–5 seconds following which the patient is instructed to completely relax. The new posterior rotation barrier is localized by further flexion of the hip joint. The mobilization is repeated 3 times.

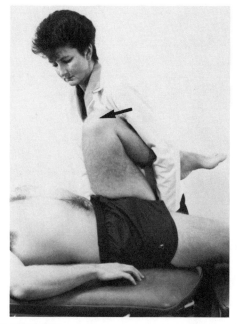

Notes:

_____

_____

_____

_____

_____

_____

_____

_____

_____

_____

_____

_____

_____

_____

_____

_____

_____

_____

_____

_____

_____

1. INNOMINATE

e) Inflare

Patient:	Supine, hip and knee on the side of the lesion flexed.
Therapist:	Standing at the patient's side.
Palpate:	With one hand, grasp the ASIS and the iliac crest of the opposite innominate. With the other hand, grasp the patient's flexed knee.
Localization:	The motion barrier is localized by abducting and externally rotating the flexed hip joint to the physiological limit. Further abduction and external rotation of the hip joint is then gently applied, while fixing the contralateral innominate, thus using the fixed hip joint as a lever to flare the lesioned innominate outwards.
Mobilization:	From this position, the patient is instructed to adduct the hip against the therapist's resistance (arrow). This isometric contraction is held for 3–5 seconds following which the patient is instructed to completely relax. The new motion barrier is localized by further abduction and external rotation of the flexed hip joint. The mobilization is repeated 3 times. Finally, the lower extremity is extended while maintaining abduction and external rotation at the hip joint.

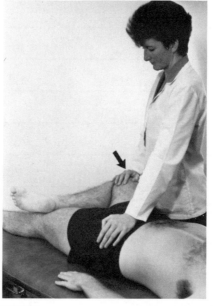

Notes:

_____

_____

_____

_____

_____

_____

_____

_____

_____

_____

_____

_____

_____

_____

_____

_____

_____

_____

_____

_____

_____

_____

_____

1. INNOMINATE

f) Outflare

Patient: Supine, hip and knee on the side of the lesion flexed.

Therapist: Standing at the patient's side.

Palpate: With the index and long fingers of the cranial hand, palpate the sacral sulcus on the side of the lesion. With the caudal hand, grasp the medial aspect of the flexed knee and cradle the lower leg against the shoulder.

Localization: The motion barrier is localized by adducting and internally rotating the flexed hip joint to the physiological limit. Further adduction and internal rotation of the hip joint is then gently applied thus using the fixed hip joint as a lever to flare the lesioned innominate inwards.

Mobilization: From this position, the patient is instructed to abduct the hip against the resistance (arrow) provided by the therapist's shoulder. This isometric contraction is held for 3–5 seconds following which the patient is instructed to completely relax. The new motion barrier is localized by further adduction and internal rotation of the flexed hip joint. The mobilization is repeated 3 times. Finally, the lower extremity is extended while maintaining adduction and internal rotation at the hip joint.

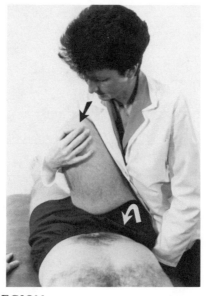

Notes:

_____

_____

_____

_____

_____

_____

_____

_____

_____

_____

_____

_____

_____

_____

_____

_____

_____

_____

_____

_____

_____

_____

1. INNOMINATE

g) Pubic Symphysis Subluxation

Patient:	Supine, hips and knees flexed.
Therapist:	Standing at the patient's side.
Palpate:	Place the hands alternately on:

a) the lateral aspect of the patient's knees, in order to resist abduction.

b) the medial aspect of the patient's knees in order to resist adduction.

Localization: None is required in this technique.

Mobilization: 'Shotgun Technique.' Initially the patient is instructed to maximally abduct the hip joints against the therapist's resistance. A 10 second isometric contraction is maintained. *Immediately,* the patient is instructed to maximally adduct the hip joints. Again an isometric contraction is maintained for 10 seconds following which the patient relaxes completely. This procedure may be repeated or an isolytic adduction contraction employed if necessary. The subluxation usually reduces during the resisted adduction phase.

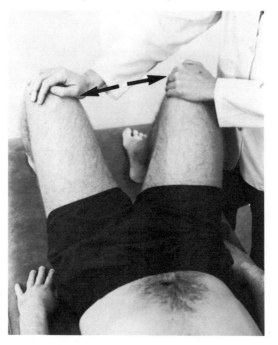

Notes:

_____

_____

_____

_____

_____

_____

_____

_____

_____

_____

_____

_____

_____

_____

_____

_____

_____

_____

_____

_____

_____

_____

2. SACRUM

a) Sacral Flexion

Patient:	Prone.
Therapist:	Standing at the patient's side.
Palpate:	With the index and long fingers of the cranial hand, palpate the sacral sulcus on the side of the lesion. With the caudal hand, support the ventral aspect of the thigh just above the knee on the side of the lesion.
Localization:	Using the caudal hand, pull the lower extremity in varying degrees of hip abduction/adduction to locate the position in which the greatest excursion of the sacroiliac joint occurs. Once located, the lower extremity is internally rotated at the hip joint and fixed by the therapist's knee. Next, place the heel of one hand over the dorsal aspect of the inferior lateral angle (ILA) on the side of the lesion. Reinforce this hand with the other. Apply a ventral force to the ILA in varying degrees of obliquity in order to determine the plane of the sacroiliac joint.
Mobilization:	This is a passive mobilization with a respiratory assist. The patient is instructed to inspire deeply during which the therapist applies a ventral force in the plane of the sacroiliac joint. Towards the end of inspiration, the patient is instructed to take three further short breaths, holding briefly between each inspiratory effort. The patient is then instructed to breath out. The ventral force on the ILA is maintained through-out the technique. The mobilization is repeated 3 times.

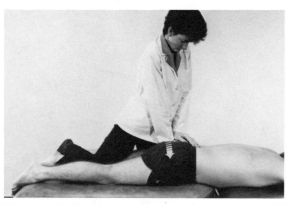

Notes:

_____

_____

_____

_____

_____

_____

_____

_____

_____

_____

_____

_____

_____

_____

_____

_____

_____

_____

_____

_____

_____

_____

_____

2. SACRUM

b) Sacral Torsion in Flexion

Patient: Sidelying on the side of the torsion (left torsion; left sidelying) with the lower arm resting behind the back, the upper arm hanging over the edge of the table. The hips and knees are comfortably flexed.

Therapist: Standing facing the patient.

Palpate and localization: With the index and long fingers of the cranial hand, palpate the L5–S1 interspace. Instruct the patient to reach towards the floor with the uppermost arm until motion is perceived at the L5–S1 joint complex. Then, with the caudal hand grip the patient's feet and support the flexed knees against the abdomen. Flex the L5–S1 joint complex fully, then return to neutral. The motion barrier of sacral torsion is then localized by allowing the feet to descend towards the floor until a firm resistance is encountered. The cranial hand palpates the sacral sulci during this manoeuvre.

Mobilization: From this position, the patient is instructed to reach towards the floor with the uppermost arm and to lift the feet towards the ceiling against the therapist's resistance (arrow). This isometric contraction is held for 3–5 seconds following which the patient is instructed to completely relax. The new motion barrier is localized by allowing the feet to descend further towards the floor. The mobilization is repeated 3 times.

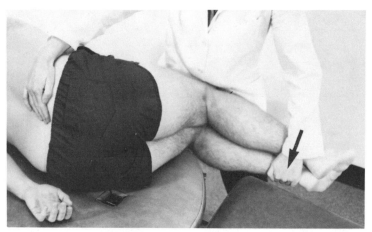

Notes:

_____

_____

_____

_____

_____

_____

_____

_____

_____

_____

_____

_____

_____

_____

_____

_____

_____

_____

_____

_____

_____

_____

2. SACRUM

c) Sacral Torsion in Extension

Patient: Standing beside the table which is level with the anterior superior iliac spines, upper body resting prone over the table, hands in a 'press up' position.

Therapist: Standing at the patient's side.

Palpate: With the ventral hand, grip the contralateral innominate bone. The forearm rests transversely across the ventral aspect of the pelvis. With the heel of the dorsal hand, palpate the sacral ILA on the side of the torsion (left torsion; left sacral ILA).

Localization: Apply a ventral force to the sacral ILA in varying degrees of obliquity in order to determine the plane of the sacroiliac joint.

Mobilization: The patient is instructed to slowly extend/rotate the lumbar spine passively by doing progressive unilateral pressups; alternating sides each time. Simultaneously, the therapist firmly 'hugs' the pelvic girdle with the ventral arm/hand and applies a ventral pressure to the sacral ILA with the dorsal hand. The obliquity of this pressure may be modified during this technique in accordance with the resistance encountered. The entire technique may be repeated if necessary.

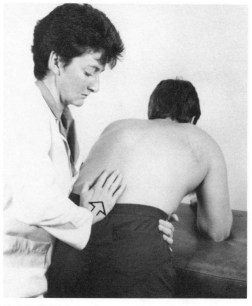

Notes:

_____

_____

_____

_____

_____

_____

_____

_____

_____

_____

_____

_____

_____

_____

_____

_____

_____

_____

_____

_____

Denise Dumonggk